Guidebook to accompany
The Better Memory Kit

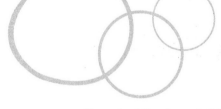

Dharma Singh Khalsa, M.D.

Copyright © 2004 by Dharma Singh Khalsa

Published and distributed in the United States by: Hay House, Inc., P.O. Box 5100, Carlsbad, CA 92018-5100 • *Phone:* (760) 431-7695 or (800) 654-5126 • *Fax:* (760) 431-6948 or (800) 650-5115 • www.hayhouse.com • **Published and distributed in Australia by:** Hay House Australia Pty. Ltd., 18/36 Ralph St., Alexandria NSW 2015 • *Phone:* 612-9669-4299 • *Fax:* 612-9669-4144 • www.hayhouse.com.au • **Published and distributed in the United Kingdom by:** Hay House UK, Ltd. • Unit 62, Canalot Studios • 222 Kensal Rd., London W10 5BN • *Phone:* 44-20-8962-1230 • *Fax:* 44-20-8962-1239 • www.hayhouse.co.uk • **Published and distributed in the Republic of South Africa by:** Hay House SA (Pty), Ltd., P.O. Box 990, Witkoppen 2068 • *Phone/Fax:* 2711-7012233 • orders@psdprom.co.za • **Distributed in Canada by:** Raincoast • 9050 Shaughnessy St., Vancouver, B.C. V6P 6E5 • *Phone:* (604) 323-7100 • *Fax:* (604) 323-2600

Editorial supervision: Jill Kramer   *Design:* Jenny Richards

All rights reserved. No part of this guidebook may be reproduced by any mechanical, photographic, or electronic process, or in the form of a phonographic recording; nor may it be stored in a retrieval system, transmitted, or otherwise be copied for public or private use—other than for "fair use" as brief quotations embodied in articles and reviews without prior written permission of the publisher. The intent of the author is only to offer information of a general nature to help you in your quest for emotional and spiritual well-being. In the event you use any of the information in this book for yourself, which is your constitutional right, the author and the publisher assume no responsibility for your actions.

Printed in China by Imago

Other Books and Audios by Dharma Singh Khalsa, M.D.

Brain Longevity (Warner Books, 1997)
The Pain Cure (Warner Books, 1999)
Meditation as Medicine
(Pocket Books—Simon & Schuster, 2001)
Food as Medicine (Atria Books—Simon & Schuster), 2003

CDs: A series of 7 CDs with Spirit Voyage Music:

First Chakra: Morning Call
Second Chakra Meditation
Meditations for the Third and Fifth Chakras
Fourth Chakra: Meditation for a Calm Heart
Sixth Chakra Meditation
Seventh and Eighth Chakras:
Meditation to Heal Self and Others
Wake Up to Wellness

• • •

Meditation for Healing: A Dialogue Between Dharma Singh Khalsa, M.D., and Deepak Chopra, M.D. (audiocassette), Hay House, 2003

• • •

In the Bliss, by Dr. Khalsa's group, Bliss, featuring Dr. D and Master L (A combination of pop/rock and inspiring words to uplift and enlighten) (© 2004 Bliss Music)

Please visit Hay House USA: **www.hayhouse.com**
Hay House Australia: **www.hayhouse.com.au**
Hay House UK: **www.hayhouse.co.uk**
Hay House South Africa: **orders@psdprom.co.za**

This project is dedicated to YB and GRD

Contents

Chapter 1:	How to Use the Guidebook, CD, and Cards	9
Chapter 2:	Why This Kit Is So Important	13
Chapter 3:	Should You Be Worried?	19
Chapter 4:	The Discovery of the Better Memory Program	25
Chapter 5:	Why the Program Works	33
Chapter 6:	The Four Pillars of Building a Better Memory	41
Chapter 7:	A Patient Regains Her Memory	45
Chapter 8:	Diet, Vitamins, and Memory-Specific Nutrients	49
Chapter 9:	*The Better Memory Kit* Mini-Cookbook	75
Chapter 10:	Stress, Meditation, and Memory	91

Chapter 11:	Exercise Lights Up Your Brain 107
Chapter 12:	The Power of Pharmaceutical Therapy........127
Chapter 13:	7 Days to a Better Memory ..145
Chapter 14:	Creating Your Own Personal Better Memory Program 179
Chapter 15:	The Final Frontier 187

Acknowledgments 191

Resources 195

About the Author 201

CHAPTER 1

How to Use the Guidebook, CD, and Cards

Congratulations and welcome! *The Better Memory Kit* is a tool that can change your life, and is based on sound science and good sense. In it I share the results of more than 12 years of study, research, and clinical experience in helping patients develop a better memory. I've worked with the past president of a foreign country, doctors, the clergy, lawyers, businesspeople, and others from all walks of life to maximize their minds, as well as prevent and reverse all types of memory loss, including Alzheimer's disease.

The kit contains this booklet you hold in

your hands for your reading and studying pleasure. It also features a powerful and enjoyable CD, which I believe is one of the main keys to the success of this program. You won't find similar material anywhere else. You'll also discover 25 memory exercise cards (plus 8 bonus cards) in the kit for effective mental exercises that I call *brain aerobics*.

Please read through the entire kit carefully before beginning the program. After you've read it through the first time, please reread it and study it. Make notes about what applies to you or your loved one's situation. And especially study Chapters 13 and 14. After that, you'll be ready to begin.

After reading the booklet the second time, please begin doing the mind/body and meditation exercises found on the CD. You'll determine the best time to do them in Chapter 14.

At the conclusion of the first seven days of the program, you'll be well on your way to having a better memory. But let me caution you about two things: The first is that to reap the benefits of the program, you must absolutely apply its principles. You can't just read about them, or only listen to the CD; you must apply the information diligently. The second is that after you start improving—and I know you will—don't stop doing the program. Keep with it, and you'll soar to new heights of mental and physical health. As many patients of mine have said: "I feel like a kid again!"

After being on the program for a while and enjoying its success, many of my patients ask: "What next?" To learn about follow-up seminars, consultations, and an outstanding interactive online support program to help you continue to build a better memory, check the Resources section at the end of this booklet.

● ● ● ● ●

CHAPTER 2

Why This Kit Is So Important

Some 4.6 million Americans currently suffer from Alzheimer's disease, the number one fear of aging people, and the worst type of memory loss. Alzheimer's causes severe damage to the nerve cells in the brain, which are called *neurons*. This results in progressive difficulty with thinking, remembering, and doing daily activities.

Because of the aging of the population, the number of Alzheimer's cases could soar to 16 million by 2050. The number of cases worldwide is expected to increase as well, perhaps reaching close to 100 million people.

The financial hardships involved with

memory loss are huge. Economists estimate that, in the United States alone, it costs at least $100 billion a year to care for people with Alzheimer's. A recent study estimated that U.S. businesses lose more than $60 billion a year because of employees who have to care for family members stricken with this disease. Moreover, businesses lose an additional, as yet undetermined, amount of money due to employees who are in the earliest stages of memory loss, and thus suffer from diminished productivity.

I say this because it's been estimated that 50 percent of people with memory loss are undiagnosed. Some working individuals may be in the early stages of memory loss without knowing it.

Memory loss has the potential to overwhelm the health-care system if nothing is done to stop it. The jump in cases could easily cause the collapse of Medicare, Medicaid, and other health-care plans that help pay for Alzheimer's care. And it almost certainly would devastate millions of American families who would have to pay for care before federal programs kick into place.

This kit offers proven strategies to prevent and reverse memory loss. It's crucial that we do so, because to delay the development of Alzheimer's by merely one year could result in a savings to society of nearly $10 billion after ten years. Moreover, to slow the beginnings of memory loss by five years would reduce the development of Alzheimer's disease by 50 percent. And slowing the onset of Alzheimer's disease by ten years, which I believe is very possible, will virtually eliminate this mind-robbing illness.

Early diagnosis and treatment are the keys to preventing and reversing Alzheimer's. No one simply wakes up with the disease: Alzheimer's begins an average of 30 years before the first symptoms appear. You read correctly—*30 years!* There are recognizable stages to the development of Alzheimer's, just as there are for many other illnesses, such as heart disease.

For example, a person with heart disease may first notice shortness of breath while exercising. Then perhaps they may develop chest discomfort, which may progress to tightness and pain radiating from the person's chest up to their neck and down their left arm. If left unrecognized and untreated, this person will go on to develop severe heart disease and possibly suffer a heart attack. Suffering a heart attack may lead to disability and perhaps a premature death.

The same goes for memory loss. A preliminary form, called mild cognitive impairment (MCI), appears before a person develops a more severe case of memory loss. The problem is that MCI progresses to Alzheimer's at a rate of 10 to 15 percent every year, which then can progress to mid-stage and late stages of the disease. Those numbers add up. That's why we must undertake a preventive strategy now.

Some Good News

I'll bet you're ready for some good news, and I have some for you. The effect of applying this program will add many years of high-functioning brain power to your life. The ultimate purpose of this kit is to help improve your memory starting right now, and to keep your mind operating at peak performance levels in the future, while preventing you from ever losing this most precious gift from your Creator.

● ● ● ● ●

CHAPTER 3

Should You Be Worried?

The short answer is . . . yes. We should all be worried because the older we get, the more likely we are to lose our memory. At age 65, for example, the incidence of Alzheimer's is 10 percent. If you're lucky enough to live to be 85, and many of us are these days, your risk of developing Alzheimer's disease is 50 percent. Moreover, if a member of your immediate family, such as your mother, father, or sibling, has had Alzheimer's, your risk increases. Genetics also play a factor: Having a gene called the ApoE4 increases your risk. But, as I'll discuss later in this booklet, there are many things you can do to prevent Alzheimer's disease, regardless of your genes. That's because memory loss is, in large measure, a disease of lifestyle. Therefore, in a manner akin to preventing heart disease, there are changes you can make to keep your mind alive well into your golden years.

Beyond age, there are other risk factors:

- Certain drugs
- Stress
- Depression
- Raised blood levels of a chemical called *homocysteine,* which can often be treated with folic acid
- Illnesses such as heart disease, anemia, or a low thyroid

A Case in Point

Marilyn knew something was seriously wrong with her 66-year-old mother when Mom forgot how to use the phone. She was also having difficulty remembering things such as words, names of familiar objects, and directions. Marilyn was also worried about *herself* because she'd started misplacing things, and would occasionally forget a word.

I explained to Marilyn that there were differences in the signs that she and her mother were displaying. The memory deficiencies Marilyn manifested were not of concern yet, but I suggested that she begin a preventive program so that her symptoms didn't worsen. Her mother's situation was more serious, however, and she was started on a program for early Alzheimer's similar to the one I'll share with you later in this kit. Within a short period of time, there was marked improvement in Mom's memory.

The 10 Warning Signs of Memory Loss

1. Forgetting things more often
2. Putting things in strange places
3. Having problems with tasks such as balancing the checkbook
4. Confusion about the date
5. Displaying a sudden change in mood or behavior
6. Difficulty finding the right words
7. Significant mood disturbances such as fear, suspicion, or confusion
8. Loss of interest in doing things
9. Forgetting common expressions or terms
10. Being confused about doing familiar things such as getting dressed

There are various stages of memory loss, and they depend on the severity and progression of the symptoms. For that reason, as I'll point out over and over again in this kit, early diagnosis and early aggressive intervention are the keys to successful treatment of memory problems. If you have no problem now, that's wonderful. But, as all the latest medical research is revealing, it's imperative that you start taking care of your brain now.

The first step, if you or a loved one is having a problem, is to visit your doctor for an evaluation, which should include a history and physical examination, laboratory tests, memory testing, and perhaps sophisticated x-rays such as a PET or SPECT scan. After you have a diagnosis, begin the Better Memory program. For further information, please check the Resources section or log on to: **www.drdharma.com**.

CHAPTER 4

The Discovery of the Better Memory Program

I began my professional medical career in anesthesiology at the University of California in San Francisco, where I was elected chief resident. In this position, I was required to participate in research and was involved in two projects. One involved the development of a new anesthetic technique for patients undergoing open-heart surgery—that study resulted in my first published paper.

Later, I was part of the research team that discovered that epidural anesthesia was the safest and most effective form of pain relief during labor and delivery. I was particularly involved in the research of epidural anesthesia during cesarean sections. Late at night and early in the morning, you could find me in the delivery suite placing epidurals and drawing the patients' blood to measure their endorphin levels, a marker of pain relief and lowered stress during anesthesia and surgery.

After my residency, I moved to New Mexico for my first position as an anesthesiologist. There a miracle happened. I met the man I recognized as my spiritual teacher—Yogi Bhajan, an enlightened yoga master. It was on Thanksgiving Day in 1981 that I received my spiritual name of Dharma Singh Khalsa. I soon learned that my name means "spiritual warrior on a victorious path." That day, I also had what I've come to call a "forward life experience." I realized that I no longer had to put people to sleep using powerful anesthetic drugs. Rather, I knew that I could now help them wake up and heal in their body, mind, and spirit by using the new healing methods I was learning.

I've used all of the knowledge that I've gained in my studies of both Western medicine and alternative or integrative medicine to create this *Better Memory Kit.*

Let me further explain the concept of integrative medicine. Imagine two rivers: The one on the left is conventional medicine, consisting of drugs and surgery; but on the right there's another river that consists of modalities found in complementary or alternative medicine. Here you'll find nutrition, vitamins, stress-management techniques such as yoga or meditation, physical exercise, and the like. When these two rivers come together in a tremendous confluence, not unlike Niagara Falls, the marvelous healing power of integrative medicine is generated.

We all have our own healing journey and our own spiritual path, and I'm no different. Change is often a slow process—after all, Rome wasn't built in a day.

MY JOURNEY TOOK MANY YEARS. I continued practicing clinical anesthesia, while at the same time I began studying holistic healing in earnest. I studied with the great, pioneering European nutritionist Paavo Airola, Ph.D. I also took basic and advanced training in mind/body medicine at Harvard Medical School under the illustrious Herbert Benson, M.D.

As my practice in anesthesiology grew into the management of complex pain problems, I decided that I needed to know more about Asian medicine if I really wanted to be of complete service to my patients. As a result of this awareness, I enrolled in the UCLA Medical Acupuncture for Physicians program. After completing this program, I developed the first holistic pain program in the Southwest at Lovelace Medical Center in Albuquerque. If you saw the movie *The Right Stuff,* then perhaps you recall that Lovelace was where the original astronauts received their physical examinations before going into outer space.

In late 1990, I was asked to become the founding director of the Acupuncture, Stress Medicine, and Chronic Pain Program at the University of Arizona's teaching hospital in Phoenix. I would become the first director of acupuncture in an American medical school. I accepted that position and created an innovative pain-medicine program, which not only helped my patients ease their chronic discomfort, but also improved their memory.

That was the beginning of the Better Memory program.

Soon I made a startling discovery. While reviewing the medical literature, I learned that chronic, unbalanced stress was very detrimental to memory function. This is because, I gleaned, stress causes the release of the hormone cortisol into the blood from our adrenal glands, which sit atop our kidneys. Cortisol, it turns out, is very toxic to our memory.

A light went on. I knew I'd made an important observation that very few people in medicine were discussing. I was, it seemed, the first practicing physician paying attention to this phenomenon.

The Alzheimer's Prevention Foundation International was created, and I moved to Tucson to begin my work helping people prevent and reverse this dreaded disease. Because I was one of the first doctors doing this work, I soon began receiving many requests for consultations. In 1995, I began my first book, *Brain Longevity,* which was published in 1997. This was the first book to put forth a program to improve the mind and memory. The rest, as they say, is history.

Over the past 12 years, I've continued my clinical work, successfully treating hundreds of patients from around the world and influencing the therapy of thousands more. Sometimes I had to deal with criticism from conventional medical doctors and organizations that persisted in their belief that nothing could be done to impact our brain. But I had patience, which I developed because I had faith in my knowledge and experience, and belief in the program that I'm about to share with you in this kit.

Dr. Dharma Goes to Washington

It was May 7, 2003. I was the first doctor to ever be invited to testify before Congress about my ideas on the prevention of Alzheimer's disease using an integrative medical approach. Afterward, I went to the Health and Human Services Building to meet the Surgeon General of the United States of America, Vice Admiral Richard Carmona, M.D., M.P.H.

In his spacious office, Dr. Carmona turned to me and said, "Your work should now be considered mainstream." With that one sentence uttered by Dr. Carmona, I felt empowered to help more people improve their memory. I was very excited to teach patients diagnosed with mild cognitive impairment (MCI) how to prevent its progression to Alzheimer's disease. I could also help more people with Alzheimer's disease slow the progression of their illness, and, in many cases, reverse their symptoms. I was thrilled that I could help others live long, happy, healthy, and productive lives.

My work, supported by the Surgeon General, made it clear to me, more than ever before, that aging need not be a time of brain degeneration, memory loss, personal pain, and financial disaster. Rather, as we age, we can develop a mind rich in wisdom, and share our experience with our children and grandchildren. Perhaps we can even do our part to make this world a better place for those who come after us.

* * * * *

CHAPTER 5

Why the Program Works

Why does my program help you build a better memory? Because, as I've said so often in my speeches and seminars: "The brain is flesh and blood, just like the rest of your body." Because the brain is flesh and blood—just like your heart, for example—it will respond to things that we can do for it. As you probably know, the heart needs adequate oxygen to flow into its muscle. It also needs other nutrients, such as B vitamins for energy. Moreover, to really work well, your heart needs exercise, which increases its blood flow and strength. Doctors also recommend stress control to prevent high blood pressure from damaging this vital organ.

All of these modalities are also vitally important for your brain and are part of *The Better Memory Kit*. The secret is that they're modified for your brain's specific use. You'll also see that there are finer points to the program, and by the end of this booklet, you'll be able to create your own personal Better Memory program, based on your own individual needs.

The Key Principle: The Brain Is Flesh and Blood

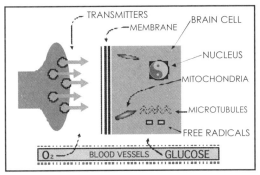

FIGURE 1

Please study the sketch of a brain cell. You can see that it is dependent upon a number of factors to function optimally. For example, the brain needs adequate blood flow, which delivers oxygen and glucose, or blood sugar, to the brain. This delivery of proper amounts of glucose is crucial to preventing and reversing memory loss, because glucose is the only fuel your brain uses. All the food you eat must first be broken down to glucose before being used by your brain.

Beyond that, your brain has to be able to build and rebuild its neurotransmitter, or brain-chemical, factory. Neurotransmitters (such as acetylcholine, your primary memory chemical) are necessary for your brain cells to send and receive messages to form new memories as well as recall old ones. There are also other neurotransmitters that are important for optimal brain function. For example, dopamine is needed for memory and mobility, a bright mood, and a lasting libido. Serotonin, the chemical increased by antidepressant drugs like Prozac, is important for happiness. Finally, other brain chemicals are needed for energy. So you see, your brain cannot function well without an adequate supply of neurotransmitters. *The Better Memory Kit* will help you maximize your neurotransmitter function.

Next, look at the outside covering of the brain cell, called the brain-cell membrane. Unfortunately, as you age, this membrane wears out, not unlike the bottom of the tires of your car. As you know, your tires don't last forever—neither does your brain-cell membrane. An important nutrient called phosphatidyl serine, which I'll discuss with you later, has been scientifically shown to preserve the stability and function of this membrane.

Now, please follow me inside the brain cell. Let's first look at the squares we call free radicals. Free radicals are actually a normal by-product of the metabolism that takes place inside your body. Oxygen, which makes up 21 percent of our inhaled air, is absolutely necessary for life. Without it, we can't last more than three minutes. Well, oxygen also leaves behind waste products, which are called free radicals. These very active chemicals can damage the insides of your cells, causing scars and a detrimental picture of accelerated aging. This may lead to inflammation, the hallmark of many chronic diseases, including Alzheimer's. The bottom line? We need to fight this free-radical damage, and many of the vitamins and brain-specific nutrients I recommend in this kit do just that.

Of course, as we've all heard: "An ounce of prevention is worth a pound of cure." As such, the program also includes simple yet powerful meditation and mind/body exercises, described both in this booklet and on the enclosed CD, to help you eliminate the dangerous stress response, which also causes the formation of free radicals.

Now let's turn our attention to the area inside the brain cell called the mitochondria. The mitochondria are your brain cells' power plant. They're responsible for creating energy through their many physiological reactions such as the Krebs cycle, which you might still remember from your chemistry or biology class as being the main way our cells function. Over the years, I've noticed that one of my patients' chief complaints is brain fatigue. A main reason for this is a fall in mitochondrial energy. In this kit, I'll share information about a very important nutrient called coenzyme Q10, which increases your mitochondrial energy. Interestingly, adequate levels of supplemental coenzyme Q10 cannot be gained from food. It's virtually impossible, even if you eat a mountain of soybeans.

Finally, let's look at the nucleus itself—this is where we find our genes and DNA. Many researchers in the field of memory believe that Alzheimer's is a genetic illness, and by finding a particular genetic twist, the disease will be cured forever. I wish they were right, but unfortunately it's simply not true. While we know that a certain genetic makeup is an important risk factor for developing Alzheimer's, it's not always the case. Some Alzheimer's victims have the genes, which impart greater risk, and some don't.

In my view, and in the view of many other forward-thinking physicians and scientists, it's the interaction of our genes with our lifestyle and environment that determines our genetic expression or outcome. It's my position that we can maintain full genetic integrity by following a lifestyle program such as the one I'm sharing with you in this kit. It's not just me saying this, either—the new and exciting developments you'll learn about in this kit are backed by solid scientific medical research on the white-hot cutting edge of medicine. And, as the Surgeon General told me in Washington, D.C., after I testified before Congress, these ideas are now becoming mainstream.

● ● ● ● ●

CHAPTER 6

The Four Pillars of Building a Better Memory

The human brain is an amazing instrument that no computer can duplicate. Believe it or not, your brain can process millions of stimuli in hundredths of a second; however, it requires good care and attention to operate at peak efficiency, especially as you enter your 40s, 50s, and beyond. So how can you take care of your brain? By following the four pillars of building a better memory:

1. Diet: I'll show you how to follow a 15 to 20 percent right-fat diet. I'll base this on the same protocol my nutritionist uses in our seminars in Tucson. In addition to the best foods for your memory, I'll also tell you about my special memory-specific nutrients.

2. Stress Reduction: As I mentioned previously, it's imperative to dissolve the stress in your life, because chronic, unbalanced pressure raises the memory-robbing chemical, cortisol, in the blood. The special meditative exercises included in this kit have been part of my clinical program for over a decade and have been found to help improve my patients' memory.

In a moment, I'll go into further detail about this very important topic, as well as teach you how to meditate. If you've never meditated before, don't worry—it's easy. I've also included meditation and mind/body exercises on the enclosed CD. On it you'll find a morning mind/body exercise and meditation I call *Energy Plus.* Then there's a second exercise for afternoon or evening use called *Tranquility Base.* I've also produced a bedtime relaxation experience for you called *Sleepy-Time Nice*. Finally, I've created a powerful visualization technique to help you consolidate the program in your mind.

3. Exercise: There are actually three types of exercises that are important to improve your memory. The first is physical exercise, such as walking and aerobic conditioning. The second is mental exercise, such as crossword puzzles and other memory-enhancing games. I'll discuss this form of thinking exercise, which I call *brain aerobics,* in great detail. In fact, it's such an important part of *The Better Memory Kit* that I've created memory exercise cards for you to incorporate into your daily activities.

Your Better Memory program will also include a powerful form of exercise for improving your memory called mind/body exercise. The Alzheimer's Prevention Foundation International, of which I am the president and medical director, has recently concluded a very innovative research project utilizing the same mind/body exercise found in this booklet and on the CD. The exercise has a very regenerating, balancing, and healing effect on the brain.

4. Pharmaceuticals: As you know by now, *The Better Memory Kit* is a medical program. For that reason, I've incorporated the most effective drugs available for preventing memory loss and slowing its progression. Beyond that, I've included the best information available on the use of hormone replacement therapy (HRT), which, as you may know, is a rather controversial area of medicine today. I believe, however, that I've researched this topic in such great detail that I can present an unbiased view on how to best use HRT to fully benefit your memory.

CHAPTER 7

A Patient Regains Her Memory

Linda was a 49-year-old worried woman from a large East Coast city. She arrived at one of my seminars in Tucson thinking that she might have early Alzheimer's. She had a family history of the disease and knew that it increased her risk. She told me that she'd suffered a gradual decline in her cognitive abilities over the past few years, especially impacting her ability to pick up complex ideas, remember names, and think of words. It was her decreased ability to remember and use words that was really bothering her, because in her position as an editor and writer, words were her stock-in-trade. She was also under a lot of stress due to the reorganization of her company, which gave her increased responsibilities.

Testing disclosed that she did indeed have a memory problem, possibly an early form of mild cognitive impairment (MCI), which may progress to Alzheimer's.

I placed Linda on a complete Better Memory program including diet; vitamins; stress-relieving meditation; and physical, mental, and mind/body exercises. I also prescribed special memory-specific nutrients and a memory-improving hormone called *pregnenolone*.

Within a week, she was going full blast on her new program and began to notice a decrease in her speech difficulties. After two months, she reported "good success" and said she was doing very well.

We adjusted her program a bit, and after another month she'd improved even more and was reporting that she'd regained her ability to find names and numbers.

This level of response is not at all unusual in people I've helped undertake a Better Memory program. Individuals with all types of memory issues—from simply wanting to improve their brain function and prevent it from declining with age to actually coping with Alzheimer's—have achieved success with the program I'm presenting in *The Better Memory Kit.*

● ● ● ● ●

CHAPTER 8

Diet, Vitamins, and Memory-Specific Nutrients

Building a better memory, preventing loss of mental function, and impacting Alzheimer's disease is, in large measure, dependent on your lifestyle, not just your genes. Since you eat so often, your diet plays a critical role in the health of your brain. People who eat a healthy diet are less likely to experience symptoms of memory loss as they age, according to medical studies. As you now know, your brain is a flesh-and-blood organ. Even so, your brain has a lot in common with a machine such as a car. Like your car, your brain needs proper fuel to work well, so you must feed your brain correctly.

One important, well-researched way to enhance one's memory is to avoid a diet high in saturated fat—such diets, based on animal products, especially red meat, are linked to inflammation and the production of free radicals. And as you know, free-radical damage may lead to the death of your brain cells.

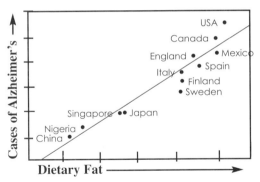

FIGURE 2

Notice that countries with the highest intake of fat, such as the United States, also have the highest incidence of Alzheimer's disease. In contrast, Asian countries, which have the lowest intake of saturated fat, have the lowest incidence of Alzheimer's. Many Asian countries such as Japan (specifically Okinawa) also enjoy the greatest longevity in the world.

Nigeria, which, of course, is not an Asian country, also has a fairly low incidence of Alzheimer's. What's their secret? The people there use low-fat grains as a major staple in their diet.

Not only do Asian countries eat a diet low in saturated fat, but they also consume high amounts of food protective against Alzheimer's disease, cardiovascular disease, and cancer. Can you guess what that food is? If you said fish, you're correct. Fish such as salmon is high in omega-3 oil or what we call "the right fat." I believe that the vast intake of fruit and vegetables, as well as the omega-3s found in fish and the vegetarian protein substitutes in the Asian diet such as soy, are protective against memory loss.

Fish oil is also on the minds of people in Washington, D.C. Citing the growth of both experimental and clinical evidence of the importance of omega-3 consumption, the White House has recently recommended these right fats in its dietary guidelines for Americans. In an interesting research project, doctors studied people from Nigeria who moved to Indiana. After living in that state for a number of years and adopting an American diet, the Nigerians' rate of Alzheimer's disease rose to meet that of people in the U.S. In another study, when Japanese people moved to America, their rate of Alzheimer's disease also rose to meet the level of Americans. These two studies highlight the impact that diet has on the development of memory loss.

A healthy diet featuring smaller portion sizes (and therefore calories), which is high in protein (but reduced in animal protein) and mixed with the right amounts of good fat and complex carbohydrates is the eating plan of choice to improve your memory, lessen your risk of Alzheimer's, and reduce the symptoms of memory loss.

The Better Memory Diet

Make your plate a multicolored rainbow. I suggest loading up on lightly steamed organic vegetables, especially spinach, and green, leafy vegetables. Broccoli and yellow turnips (rutabagas) are also beneficial, as are carrots.

All fruit is great to eat because it contains an abundance of free-radical-fighting compounds. Blueberries are particularly good memory fruits because they've been shown to protect your brain cells from degenerating. Eating a half cup of fresh or frozen organic blueberries two or three times a week is excellent for your brain.

Better Memory Fruits
(choose organic whenever possible)

- Avocados
- Cranberries
- Prunes
- Oranges
- Kiwi
- Blueberries
- Plums
- Strawberries
- Raspberries
- Red Grapes
- Blackberries

Better Memory Vegetables
(choose organic whenever possible)

- Beets
- Spinach
- Broccoli
- Kale
- Green Chilis
- Cauliflower
- Brussel Sprouts
- Red Bell Peppers

Good Fats, Bad Fats, and Your Brain

Good Fats (rich in omega-3)

Salmon	Brazil Nuts
Herring	Soy and Tofu
Sardines	Flaxseed Oil
Cashews	Pistachios
Olive Oil	Free-Range Chicken
Avocados	Lean Free-Range Meats
Anchovies	Tuna

Bad Fats (high in omega-6)

Lamb	Ice Cream
Steak	Margarine
Butter	Whole Milk
Bacon	Fried Foods
Cheese	Processed Foods
Doughnuts	

I suggest that you replace the high-fat red meat in your diet with reduced-fat free-range beef, as well as free-range chicken. Fish and soy should be eaten regularly as well. For patients with MCI, early Alzheimer's, or those who are further along in their disease process, salmon and tuna are the best fish to eat. One must be cautious, however, because of mercury issues with tuna and other concerns about farm-raised salmon, which has been shown to contain 60 times more contaminants than the fresh variety. For these reasons, I advise that you stick to fresh-frozen Alaskan salmon and avoid farmed salmon.

Besides animal products, there are other great sources of protein. Soy is an example. The creative folks in the natural-foods industry now offer a wide variety of soy products dressed up to resemble regular meat. You can find soy burgers, ground soy (which resembles hamburger), and even soy steak. There's also soy ham, turkey, and salami. Additionally, the familiar-looking white block of tofu is quite tasty when cooked with vegetables and spices. For variety, if you enjoy the taste of Indian food, try adding curry dishes to your diet. Curry contains turmeric, which has profound antioxidant properties.

In addition to avoiding excess saturated fat, another important idea behind the Better Memory diet is to keep your blood sugar stable. Following the Better Memory diet will help you maintain a high level of mental energy because it prevents you from developing low blood sugar or hypoglycemia. What I most want you to avoid is the "roller-coaster" effect caused by eating too many high-sugar foods. Roller-coaster foods are those that put your body in an alarm state, and cause too much stress on your system. It's that stress that causes injury to the memory cells in your brain. Foods that fall into the category of high-sugar alarm foods are almost all white. Examples are: sugar, bread, flour, cake, pasta, milk, white rice, and processed foods. Other examples are: soft drinks, caffeine, and excessive alcohol consumption.

This diet recommends foods and beverages that are converted slowly to sugar once they're digested and in your bloodstream. Please consult the following chart to find out which foods are relatively slow to convert to glucose. Notice, for example, that potatoes are converted to glucose more quickly than table sugar. Orange juice, in contrast, is actually converted to glucose at a slower rate.

As you can see, all foods high in fruit sugar, or fructose, are relatively slow to convert to glucose. For this reason, I recommend fructose as a sweetener, which can be bought in any health-food grocery store such as Whole Foods Market, instead of sugar or any artificial sweetener.

Sugar Chart

(Glucose, which is sugar, is 100 points, meaning that it is most rapidly converted to sugar in the blood. The lower the number, the slower the food is converted to glucose, and hence the more stable your blood sugar. This is because glucose releases insulin, which lowers blood sugar; which then causes you to feel hungry, tired, and unable to think straight.)

Glucose	100	Spaghetti	50
Potatoes	98	Orange Juice	46
Carrots	92	Grapes	45
Honey	87	Apples	39
White Rice	72	Yogurt	36
White Bread	69	Tofu	35
Brown Rice	66	Milk	34
Bananas	62	Grapefruit	26
Sucrose (table sugar)	59	Fructose	20

The delicious recipes in the next chapter all follow the principles of the Better Memory diet. They are low in fat, high in protein, and rich in natural, memory-enhancing vitamins and minerals.

Alcohol and Your Memory

Research has shown that drinking one to two glasses of wine or spirits a few times a week can help prevent dementia by up to 70 percent. Why is that? In the first place, alcohol helps thin your blood, preventing clogging of vessels; it also increases your good cholesterol. In addition, according to one study, drinking a moderate amount of alcohol may increase acetylcholine, the memory chemical. Drinking red wine has a beneficial effect because it contains resveratrol, a powerful antioxidant.

So, is all this good news? The answer is in your hands. You simply have to decide if you want alcohol consumption to be a regular part of your lifestyle. Remember: The normal amount of alcohol in your blood, and hence your brain, is zero. Any amount you add can therefore be considered a toxin—I've seen many patients in whom alcohol consumption got out of control and caused brain damage.

You also should know that many of the positive effects of moderate alcohol consumption could be replicated by other means. For example, exercise, eating a good diet, and stress control all convey the same benefits.

If you can control your drinking, then enjoying a couple of glasses of wine or a cocktail periodically, but not daily, can reduce your chance of developing dementia.

Vitamins and Memory-Specific Nutrients

Conventional medicine primarily approaches the prevention and reversal of memory loss by looking for an ever-elusive magic-bullet drug. I've been able to help many people improve their memory and reverse memory loss with the following nutrients.

First of all, everyone should take a high-potency multiple vitamin and mineral capsule such as my *Longevity Gold Caps.*

Be sure to compare the ingredients

contained in the *Longevity Gold Caps* with other products sold at drugstores and advertised on television as being complete and high potency. You'll notice a big difference. The *Longevity Gold Caps* have every vitamin and mineral you'll ever need to build a better memory at correct dosages, including folic acid, which, as I mentioned previously, is important because it decreases a chemical in your blood called homocysteine. Homocysteine is a risk factor for both heart disease and memory loss. *The Longevity Gold Caps* also contain sufficient amounts of the powerful antioxidant vitamin C, which has been shown to reduce the risk of Alzheimer's disease by 20 percent when taken with vitamin E. (The dose of vitamin C should be at least 2,000 mg per day.)

Now let's consider the chief memory-specific nutrients:

- **Vitamin E:** Fights free radicals
- **Coenzyme Q10:** Increases energy
- **Ginkgo Biloba:** Enhances blood flow
- **Phosphatidyl Serine (PS):** Regenerates brain-cell membranes
- **DHA:** Supports focus and concentration.

— **Vitamin E:** Vitamin E, or tocopherol, is a potent antioxidant that protects the brain from free-radical damage. It may reduce the risk of Alzheimer's by 36 percent and slow the progression of even mid-stage Alzheimer's. I recommend taking a mixed form of alpha and gamma tocopherol for:

- *Prevention and better memory:* 400 IU once or twice per day
- *Mild cognitive impairment (MCI):* 1,000 IU once or twice per day
- *Alzheimer's disease:* 1,000 IU twice per day

— Take Coenzyme Q10 for:

- *Prevention and energy:* 100 mg per day
- *Memory loss:* 300 mg per day

As you can see by studying the graph below, Coenzyme Q10 decreases in your brain with age. Moreover, it's impossible to obtain enough Coenzyme Q10 in your diet to replenish it. As it is needed for brain-cell energy production, it must be taken as a supplement.

FIGURE 3

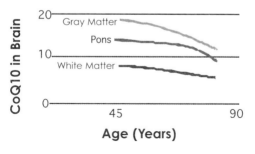

Recent clinical research reveals that patients with memory loss from Parkinson's disease may benefit from 1,200 mg of Coenzyme Q10, especially when combined with at least 100 mg of alpha-lipoic acid, an important cell nutrient.

There's one other case that's important to mention. Those of you taking statin cholesterol-lowering medication must supplement with Coenzyme Q10. Statins deplete your cells of this all-important energy compound, which is the reason that one of the main side effects of the drug is severe muscle pain, sometimes leading to muscle-cell death and kidney failure, which can be fatal. The dose is 300 mg per day.

— **Ginkgo Biloba:** Gingko improves brain blood flow and fights free radicals. It's an excellent herb to tone your brain. In my experience, it does improve memory, even in a person with minimal decline, as well as helping patients with all types of memory loss, including Alzheimer's. I suggest taking Ginkgo Biloba for:

- *Prevention and better memory:* 120 mg per day
- *MCI and Alzheimer's:* 240 mg per day

— Phosphatidyl serine (PS): Many excellent studies show PS to be successful in reversing memory loss. Name-finding, number recall, and face recognition are all improved. According to one leading researcher, PS may reverse brain aging by as much as 12 years. I recommend it for:

- *Prevention and better memory:* 100 mg per day
- *MCI:* 200 mg per day
- *Alzheimer's:* 300 mg per day

— **DHA:** DHA is a powerful omega-3 oil derived from algae. It supports optimal brain function, especially helping with focus and concentration. Anyone concerned about their memory should take omega-3 supplements for:

- *All types of memory concerns:* 500–1,000 mg per day (see below for special circumstances)

A remote side effect of taking vitamin E, DHA, and Gingko together is possible blood-thinning. Discuss this with your doctor. I haven't seen any problem with this combination of nutrients, but I do suggest that you stop taking it four days before any scheduled surgical procedure.

Secondary Nutrients

   — **Acetyl-L-Carnitine (ALC):** *Up to 2,000 mg per day.* ALC is useful because it increases brain-cell energy. It does this by acting in the mitochondria, your brain-cell power plant. ALC is particularly effective in younger patients, in whom it improves memory, word-finding, and attention.

   — **Alpha-Lipoic Acid (ALA):** *100 mg–300 mg twice per day.* I consider ALA an important nutrient for brain-cell protection, especially when taken together with Coenzyme Q10. ALA is gaining a tremendous amount of support from leading scientists and doctors because it enhances the activity of other antioxidants, most notably vitamins C and E. Moreover, ALA increases the activity of the most important antioxidant inside your cells, glutathione.

These are the most important memory-specific nutrients. Because I've seen many patients who have difficulty finding the appropriate formulations of these nutrients, I've designed two combination brain products I call *The Longevity Brain Tabs* and *The Longevity Energy Caps.* The former contains PS, Ginkgo, and DHA in one capsule, while the latter contains Coenzyme Q10, ALA, and ALC. They're very easy to use, and they save time and money because they're formulated together.

Special Supplements for Mild Cognitive Impairment (MCI) and Alzheimer's

If a patient of mine has developed mild cognitive impairment or Alzheimer's disease, I utilize the following advanced nutrients in addition to those described above. My third brain compound, *The Longevity Memory Caps,* contains the first two nutrients.

1. Huperzine A: *50–100 mg twice per day.* Huperzine A is derived from Chinese club moss and is very helpful in treating MCI and Alzheimer's. It strengthens overall brain function and improves short-term memory by increasing the amount of brain cell acetylcholine.

2. Vinpocetine: *2.5–5 mg twice per day.* Vinpocetine is derived from the periwinkle plant. It increases brain circulation and energy.

3. Galantamine: *4–8 mg per day.* According to legend, Galantamine is the same memory function enhancer used 3,200 years ago by the Greek hero Odysseus, the champion of memory and the enemy of forgetfulness. Galantamine is a plant extract, or phytonutrient, which comes from the common snowdrop, daffodil, and spider lily, among other plants. It increases the level of your two important memory-improving chemicals.

Galantamine, in its natural form, is worth

trying in cases of mild memory loss or for prevention and memory enhancement. I usually recommend using Memantine, a drug synthesized from Galantamine, if a patient has Alzheimer's disease. Memantine, which I'll discuss later in this booklet, is proving effective in mid- to late-stage Alzheimer's disease.

Please consult the charts in Chapter 13 to determine the correct program for you or your loved one.

Special Circumstances

Adult Attention Deficit Disorder (ADD), Chronic Fatigue, Chemo-Brain

In addition to prescribing the above memory-specific nutrients for people suffering with these problems, I recommend taking my *Longevity Green Drink* daily. This supplement contains plant extracts, which include important trace elements that are rapidly absorbed into your blood and go directly to your brain to help to increase your focus, attention, and concentration. *The Longevity Green Drink* wakes up your brain. In addition to helping people with the following unique circumstances, it's also very popular with people wanting to enhance their normal memory or gain more mental energy, and in patients with MCI and Alzheimer's.

DHA and Attention Deficit

DHA, fish oil, and flaxseed oil are quite helpful in restoring top levels of concentration. Here are my recommended doses:

- **DHA:** 500–1,000 mg per day
  or
- **Fish Oil:** 500–1,000 mg per day
  or
- **Flaxseed Oil:** 500–1,000 mg per day

Arginine and Vascular Dementia

A lack of blood flow to your brain cells is one cause of memory loss. Following all the steps discussed up to this point will help prevent vascular dementia; but there's one additional nutrient to mention—arginine.

Arginine is an amino acid or a protein building block that increases a chemical called *nitric oxide* (not *nitrous* oxide or laughing gas), which causes your blood vessels to widen. Under certain conditions, such as vascular disease, your body needs more arginine than is found in your diet, so supplementation is necessary. The best way to get this nutrient is by taking a specially formulated effervescent powder called *Herc Vitality Drink Mix*. You simply mix one packet in water and drink it up to three times a day.

You can find more information about all of the nutrients and supplements mentioned in this chapter, as well as purchase them, at **www.drdharma.com**, or by calling (888) 234-0459.

☆ ☆ ☆ ☆ ☆

CHAPTER 9

The Better Memory Kit Mini-Cookbook

The Better Memory Breakfast
(Makes 1 serving)

1 cup of nonfat organic yogurt
½–1 tablespoon lemon juice,
 according to taste
⅓ cup bottled water
½ scoop of *The Longevity Green Drink*
Optional: ½ organic apple or banana

Place all ingredients in blender, liquefy, and drink as your first meal of the day. Yogurt provides protein and probiotic, or friendly, intestinal bacteria; while the green powder provides easily digestible trace elements and minerals. Overall, this juice is an excellent brain-function enhancer. Fresh juices are best consumed within 2–3 hours of preparation and should be refrigerated.

The Better Memory Smoothie
(Makes 1 serving)

1 cup unsweetened pineapple juice
   (canned is okay)
½ scoop of *The Longevity Green Drink*
1 scoop of non-GMO soy or
   whey protein powder
½ cup organic blueberries

Wash and dry blueberries. Place them in a blender together with all other ingredients, liquefy, and drink as your first meal of the day. This drink is powerful and only contains 300 calories. Protein powder will give you stamina to face the day; the green powder provides trace elements and minerals; the pineapple juice is excellent as a digestion aid, diuretic, and fat burner; and the blueberries are a specific brain tonic.

Dr. Dharma's Energy Cocktail
(Makes 1 serving)

1 cup unsweetened pineapple juice
  (canned is okay)
½ papaya
2 fresh apricots
½ mango
½ cup ice
Water as needed
Optional: Add ¼ scoop of *The Longevity Green Drink* and/or 1 scoop of non-GMO soy or whey protein powder.

Wash and dry the papaya, apricots, and mango. Peel and take the seeds out of the papaya, peel and pit the mango, and take pits out of the apricots. Place all ingredients in a blender, liquefy, and drink. These fruits contain high amounts of minerals, vitamins, and fiber, which are very beneficial for keeping healthy skin, circulation to all the internal organs, good vision, and proper digestion. Fresh juices are best consumed within 2–3 hours of preparation and should be refrigerated.

Fruit Salad Cocktail
(Makes 1 serving)

1 medium bunch grapes
½ apple
¼ lemon, peeled

Wash and dry ingredients, and combine them in a juicer; blend. The Fruit Salad Cocktail provides good amounts of antioxidants, vitamins, and minerals that help concentration and optimal brain function. Fresh juices are best consumed within 2–3 hours of preparation and should be refrigerated.

The Rainbow Plate
(Makes 4 servings)

4 small beets, peeled and sliced
2 cups broccoli florets
2 cups kale
½ cup edamame
2 teaspoons garlic, minced
⅓ onion, chopped
1 teaspoon ginger, minced
2 teaspoons extra-virgin olive oil
4 veggie burgers

Dressing:
½ cup low-fat cottage cheese
1 tablespoon tahini paste
1 clove garlic
2 tablespoons lemon juice
2 teaspoons Bragg Liquid Aminos
1 tablespoon parsley
¼ teaspoon sea salt
1 tablespoon bottled water

Wash and dry all ingredients, then put beets in a steamer and cook for 20 minutes or until soft. Add the broccoli, kale, and edamame and cook for 5–8 more minutes. In the meantime, sauté onion, garlic, ginger, and olive oil for 3 minutes, or until light brown. Add the veggie burgers and cook for 2–3 minutes, then flip them and cook for another 2–3 minutes. If the pan becomes sticky, add a little water. In a food processor, blend all dressing ingredients until smooth. Serve on individual plates with the veggie burger in the middle and the vegetables arranged all around it.

Drizzle 2 tablespoons of dressing per plate on top of the vegetables.

The rainbow plate is an important example of the ideal way to eat for your body and your mind. All of these vegetables provide antioxidants, phytonutrients, fiber, and trace elements necessary to slow the aging process. Experiment with different vegetables to create a rainbow on your plate!

Omega Mind Dinner
(Makes 4 servings)

2 medium baking potatoes
Four 5- to 6-oz. boneless,
    skinless salmon fillet steaks
1 cup broccoli florets
1 cup carrots, sliced
1 cup spinach, chopped

Dressing:
Makes ¼ cup

4 teaspoons extra-virgin olive oil
½ teaspoon garlic
¼ teaspoon black pepper
2 teaspoons Bragg Liquid Aminos
1 teaspoon lemon juice
½ teaspoon thyme
1 tablespoon water

Wash and dry potatoes, then prick the skins to allow steam to escape. Wrap each one in aluminum foil and bake at 375° for 45–55 minutes or until soft when pierced with a fork. Broil the salmon fillets for 5 minutes, then turn them over and broil for 5 more minutes, or until salmon is cooked throughout. Time may vary according to thickness of steak. Let salmon cool for 5 minutes then cut into long strips. Steam carrots for 5 minutes, then add broccoli and cook for another 5 minutes. Finally, add spinach and steam for another 2 minutes.

To serve, cut the potatoes in half and place each half on an individual dinner plate. Divide the vegetables among the plates, and arrange the salmon strips on top of the vegetables. In a small bowl, whisk all dressing ingredients together, pour over dinner plate, and serve.

Salmon contains omega-3 oils, which are very important for a better memory; carrots, broccoli, and spinach also support brain function with their high antioxidant content.

Protein Surprise
(Makes 4 servings)

1 package of firm tofu (about 16 oz.)
2 teaspoons extra-virgin olive oil
¼ cup soy sauce or Bragg Liquid Aminos
¼ cup bottled water
1 tablespoon peeled and finely grated ginger
1 clove garlic, finely minced
Juice of 1 lemon

Rinse and cut tofu in half-inch slices. Combine olive oil, soy sauce, ginger, garlic, and lemon juice in the bottom of a glass baking pan. Add the tofu and let marinate for 2–3 hours, flipping tofu once while marinating. Then bake at 350º for 30 minutes. If the marinade evaporates completely and tofu starts sticking, simply add a little water. Serve with sautéed or steamed vegetables.

Tucson Power Plate (TPP)
(Makes 8 servings)

I absolutely love this meal. It's a delicious, nutritious dish that's high in complete protein, low in bad fat, and contains an acceptable amount of carbohydrates for usable and sustained energy. This is one dish where you can eat as much as you like and not gain weight. The reason? It's easily digested and seems to increase your metabolism. Medically speaking, I suggest the TPP for patients who are recovering from an illness or are in a weakened condition for some reason. The TPP is a very simple food combination that's also quite cleansing for both the body and mind.

1 cup mung beans
10 cups water
1-inch piece of kombu seaweed
1 cup white basmati rice
1 teaspoon Bragg Liquid Aminos per serving
1 teaspoon extra-virgin olive oil per serving

Soak beans overnight. Wash beans and rice. Bring water to boil, add beans and kombu seaweed, and let boil over medium-high heat for approximately 45–50 minutes until soft. Then add the rice and let simmer for another 20–25 minutes until well done. Add Bragg or soy sauce to taste. You can also add one teaspoon of extra-virgin olive oil per person. Eat with salad and/or steamed vegetables. (For smaller quantities, reduce the amount of mung beans and rice.)

Spectacular Tofu Salad

(Makes 4 servings)

1 package of firm tofu (about 16 oz.)
Juice of 1 lemon
3 celery sticks, finely diced
⅔ cup grated radishes, carrots, and zucchini
½ sweet red pepper, finely chopped
2–3 dill pickles, finely chopped

Dressing:
¼–½ cup eggless, sugarless mayonnaise
   (from natural-food stores)
2–3 tablespoons prepared mustard
1 teaspoon lemon juice
½ teaspoon sea salt
½ teaspoon black pepper

Rinse and cut tofu in half-inch slices. Sprinkle with lemon juice, and bake in a lightly oiled baking dish at 375° until medium hard, about 20 to 25 minutes. Let cool, then grate it.

Meanwhile, in a mixing bowl, combine celery, radishes, carrots, zucchini, red pepper, and pickles. Add the grated tofu to the rest of ingredients and mix well. The texture of the grated, baked tofu in this dish is similar to chicken or tuna salad. In a small bowl, mix all dressing ingredients and add to the salad. Serve with crackers or with lettuce on bread.

The Perfect Memory Meal
(Makes 4 servings)

Salad:
4 cups mixed greens
2 tablespoons mixed raw nuts
2 tablespoons raisins
1 cup baked tofu, chopped

Dressing:
3 teaspoons extra-virgin olive oil
¼ cup orange juice
2 teaspoons Bragg Liquid Aminos

Toss the salad in a mixing bowl. In a separate bowl, whisk all the dressing ingredients. Toss salad with dressing and serve.

Main Course: *Spinach Surprise*
2 teaspoons extra-virgin olive oil
3 cloves garlic, minced
3 green onions, chopped
1 cup mushrooms, chopped
2 bunches spinach
¼ teaspoon sea salt and pepper
2 tablespoons lemon juice
1½ tablespoons grated romano
   or parmesan cheese

Lightly coat a skillet with olive oil. Sauté garlic, green onions, and mushrooms for 3–5 minutes. Fill skillet with thoroughly washed and chopped spinach. Add salt, pepper, and lemon. Cook with lid on for 2–3 minutes. Sprinkle with grated romano or parmesan cheese and serve.

Dessert: *Apple Crumble*
(Makes 6 servings)

5 medium apples, peeled and sliced thin
⅓ cup honey
Juice of ½ lemon, about 2 tablespoons
1 teaspoon grated lemon rind
½ teaspoon cinnamon
⅛ teaspoon nutmeg
1 tablespoon melted butter or ghee
1 cup granola
1 cup apple juice
Optional: ½ cup raisins, ¼ cup mixed nuts (chopped)

Place the apples, honey, lemon juice and rind, and cinnamon in a mixing bowl and stir to combine. Spread in an 8-inch baking dish. In a separate bowl, combine butter and granola and spread over apples, then add the apple juice to provide moisture for cooking. Bake at 350º for 40 minutes. May be served with ½ cup of nonfat vanilla yogurt per person.

* * * * *

CHAPTER 10

Stress, Meditation, and Memory

Did you know that being prone to psychological distress could destroy your memory and cause Alzheimer's disease? Well, as all my research shows, it can.

Have you ever been over your stress limit? At one time or another, almost all of us have. Especially since September 11, 2001, doctors and health officials have come to realize how heavy a toll stress is taking on our health. In my experience, close to 100 percent of patients have stress-related symptoms. A testimony to that is the fact that tranquilizers, antidepressants, high blood-pressure medicines, and antacids—all of which are used for illnesses made worse by stress—are the best-selling drugs on Earth.

So what is stress? At our seminars I always ask the attendees to please take a moment to think about the answer to this question. Each person's response is different. To some, the answer may be the symptoms they feel when they're under pressure in some way. An example of that might be: "Stress is when I get a headache or a stomachache." For others, stress may be a feeling: "It's when I feel jumpy or nervous."

The best definition of stress I've found is depicted in Figure 4.

FIGURE 4

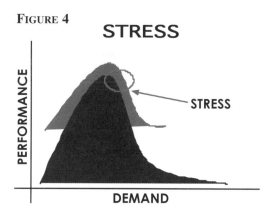

Please observe the graph. Can you see a line across the bottom called *demand* and a line going up and down called *performance?* As you examine the graph, you'll notice that, as demand increases, so does performance. Up to a certain point, that is. Notice that when our ability to perform is exceeded by the demand placed upon us, our performance drops. This increase in demand can be conscious or not—in other words, we don't even have to know about it. Thus, when our ability to perform is exceeded by the demand, known or unknown—conscious or not—we have too much stress and our performance goes down.

At that moment, we also release stress chemicals in our body, such as adrenaline, which is responsible for our fast heart rate and that alert feeling. We also release cortisol, which, as I mentioned before, seeks out and destroys the cells in the brain's memory center. Cortisol turns the memory center into a toxic dump, killing brain cells by the thousands. The problem is that as we age or develop an illness, we have a decreased ability to handle stress and lower blood cortisol levels. Cortisol wreaks havoc on our memory center: It stops glucose from entering our brain cells, it blocks our neurotransmitter function, and it causes brain cells to become injured and die. This happens because cortisol also allows the number of free radicals in the brain to skyrocket. One of the best things about *The Better Memory Kit* is that it will help save brain cells by dramatically lowering cortisol levels.

The effects of stress and cortisol on memory function have been well studied. As stress and cortisol levels increase, so does the chance of developing memory loss. This memory loss begins with a drop in the ability to recall information that we already know, such as a friend's phone number. It also impacts our ability to learn and retain new information. When this becomes a problem, it's called *short-term memory loss*. We see this when someone repeats the same story over and over again, or when a person knows very well where they went to high school and what happened many years ago, yet can't remember what they had for lunch today. As this progresses and more brain cells die, the problem worsens to the point where the individual may not be able to retain much information at all. They may lose track of dates and places. Quite often, a victim of Alzheimer's may become lost very easily.

However, memory loss doesn't have to be that severe to be significant. I recall a

41-year-old executive in the food business who complained of not being able to "keep my arms around everything anymore." His work was suffering, and he was living in fear of developing progressive memory loss. Happily, after following the Better Memory program, especially the meditation and mind/body exercises, he regained an almost perfect memory and youthful mind.

There are very few people who can actually reduce their responsibilities; in fact, busy people are probably the least able to cut back. I'm often reminded of the old adage, "If you want something done, whom do you ask?" The answer, of course, is "a busy person." Actually, I've amended this saying somewhat to now read: "If you want something done, ask a busy woman." Women often seem to be the busiest people around and the hardest hit by stress. Not coincidentally, they also have the highest incidence of Alzheimer's.

Even retirees have increased demands on them in these very busy times. Financial issues, medical problems, and family concerns take up a lot of time and energy. Beyond that, almost everyone these days is worried about the state of the world, the chance of terrorism, and their own safety.

Wouldn't it be wonderful if we could find some way to shift the curve up and to the left? In other words, if for the same demand we were actually able to increase our performance. That's where meditation fits in the picture. Meditation increases our ability to perform by reducing stress, thus lowering cortisol and improving many aspects of mental function. This adjusts the curve in the way I've mentioned. Of course, meditation has other benefits as well. In research studies over three decades, meditation has been shown to help your heart, reduce anxiety, lessen chronic pain, and increase longevity. (Please consult my book *Meditation as Medicine* to learn more about meditation's many healthful and spiritual effects.)

Further on in this booklet, I'll ask you to

plug my various recommendations into your lifestyle using a daily activities chart. One of the activities you'll use is basic meditation, primarily in the afternoon. I'll also ask you to practice my special mind/body exercise routine in the morning.

What follows are instructions in basic meditation. Even if you already know how to meditate, please read this section anyway. It's always good to review.

How to Meditate

We have three usual or normal states into which we all enter every day: *the awake state, the sleep state,* and *the dream state.* To enter into a fourth state, or *the self-healing meditative state,* requires action. Here are the four steps needed to enter into the meditative state:

1. Comfort: You don't have to sit like a pretzel to meditate. In fact, in our seminars we meditate in soft chairs. One caveat is that you don't want to be so comfortable that you fall asleep. The reason is that sleep and meditation are different states—you actually get a deeper rest with meditation.

2. Quiet: Meditation time is a special time, not to be interrupted by the telephone, fax machine, or pets. And please turn off your cell phone—your time to meditate is sacred. If your spouse or significant other doesn't meditate, they shouldn't be in the room with you. The same holds true for children.

3. A Tool: In the basic form of meditation, your tool can be any thought, sound, short prayer, or phrase that you wish to focus on during meditation. It can really be anything. Even paying attention to your breath works well. Ideally, your word should be something easy, like *peace, love, heal,* or *one,* which has a long history of being used in the research on basic meditation.

You can use any word you want, however. A very successful businessman I once taught to meditate chose the word *computer*. An anesthesiologist selected the name of his favorite drug, *Halothane*. The word you choose should be something positive, however. So, for most people, *alimony* is probably not a good choice.

Some words are more powerful than others. In a research project at Harvard Medical School, for example, the yoga sounds of *Sat Nam* on the inhale and *Wha Hey Guru* on the exhale were shown to directly activate the memory area of the brain. I'll delve into the reasons behind that more deeply in the section on mind/body exercise.

4. An Attitude: Once you begin to meditate, you'll be surprised to discover that your mind reacts like a four-year-old child. If you ask small children to sit still, they'll probably end up running all around the room. It's the same with your mind—when you expect it to calm down, it will actually speed up. Why is this so? Well, all the pressure we have stored inside our mind for our entire life is pent up in there, so when we begin to meditate, it's as if a trap door opens and "Boom!"—all these thoughts come flying out:

"Why didn't I go to the bathroom before I started?"
"I have to balance my checkbook."
"I sure hope we get that loan."
"Where's my brother? He was supposed to be here an hour ago."
"Whatever happened to Joan from the first grade?"
"What are we going to have for dinner tonight?"

When you meditate, your mind will be bombarded by thoughts. I've been meditating for three decades, and it still happens to me every day. Not to worry: This is simply the process of meditation, and it's normal and expected. It's what you do with these thoughts that really counts. And what you should do is just let them go and return to your word. As one of my patients from England once said, in a great Beatles accent, "Oh, Dr. Dharma. You mean you just start all over again?" That's right. When other thoughts enter your mind, you just start all over again. The way you do that is by going back to your focus word. For example, let's say your word is *one*. When other thoughts enter your mind, you simply say to yourself: "Oh, well, [your name], relax, one." That's all there is to it. It's easy.

A Few Words about Prayer

Prayer, as many of you might agree, is a beautiful way to create and enjoy a connection with our Higher Power. It's also most beneficial for our mental, physical, and spiritual health. When it comes to entering the fourth state, your prayer needs to be short and repetitive. You can pick a part of your favorite psalm, for example, and repeat it. You can say, "The Lord is my Shepherd," "Our Father Who Art in Heaven," "Jesus loves me," "Shalom," "Shema Yisrael," or any short prayer you desire. It just shouldn't engage your intellect, because then you'll be taken out of the fourth state.

Timing

As I will present to you on the CD, the basic meditation should last at least ten minutes. You'll design your own Better Memory program in a later section of this booklet, and then you'll discover the best time for you to meditate. Generally, I recommend practicing the mind/body exercises presented in the next section in the morning, and the basic meditation in the late afternoon or early evening.

Meditation and Your Spirit

One of the more interesting avenues of research on meditation recently has been to explore how meditation impacts our brain, and specifically how meditation changes the brain's anatomy when we have a spiritual experience. What we've learned is that when we enter the fourth state, the left side of our brain decreases in activity. In other words, there's a spot in our brain that, when stimulated during meditation, elicits a spiritual experience that allows us to feel close to God. Beyond that, many positive health benefits ensue, including better medical outcomes when an intervention such as surgery is needed. Along the way, meditating develops many positive psychological health characteristics within us, such as forgiveness, compassion, and empathy that are useful to us, our family, the community, and the world.

Philosophers and religious scholars are now debating this finding. Is God simply a product of the stimulation of this spot, some ask? Others say, "No, the Creator put this spot in our brain so we could have the experience of realizing His presence within ourselves." What do *you* think?

● ● ● ● ●

CHAP

Exercise Lights Up Your Brain

You don't have to be an Olympic athlete to exercise and live a healthy lifestyle. When you work out regularly, research shows that you have a better-functioning memory. To maintain a high level of stamina in your daily life requires mental energy. Exercise increases that as well.

The exercises prescribed in *The Better Memory Kit* can be divided into three distinct and important types: physical, mental, and mind/body. Let's start with physical exercise.

Importance of Physical Exercise

Physical exercise is imperative because it reduces your risk of developing Alzheimer's disease by 50 percent, according to research. Moreover, women who engaged in a regular exercise program from ages 40 to 60 show a dramatic reduction in cognitive decline. Regular physical exercise increases brain blood flow, improves the biochemistry of your brain, and regenerates brain cells. Exercise also lowers high blood pressure, which is a risk factor for memory loss.

All my seminars include a strong exercise section. I recommend at least 30 minutes of aerobic exercise and weight training three to four times a week to promote cardiovascular and brain fitness. Lower-intensity activities such as walking are beneficial as well. I usually prescribe brisk walking for a time period of 30 minutes, three or four times a week. Walking reduces stress, increases your mental energy level, and helps you remain trim.

One patient of mine, a 66-year-old woman with early memory loss, was not in the habit of exercising. In her case, I simply suggested that she start by opening her front door and walking for about ten minutes and then turning around and walking back. She did that, and really began to enjoy her exercise program, which I'm sure contributed to her memory improvement.

What about the person with Alzheimer's disease? He or she can walk outside with a caregiver, around an outdoor courtyard, or even inside with assistance, if needed.

Besides simply opening the door and going outside, there are some other ways to bring walking into your life. One is to exercise for a short period of time. For example, park a block away from your destination and walk the difference. You can also walk to the store, if possible, or around the mall.

There are many other ways to exercise. One of my favorites is playing tennis. The great thing about tennis is that it's fun.

Regardless of your age or ability, you can always hit with a teaching pro or take a lesson. My tennis teacher, Britt Feldhausen, an award-winning, certified teaching professional, told me that, in his extensive experience, very few tennis players develop Alzheimer's disease. I believe the reason tennis gives you such a high level of mental fitness is because playing the game engages your mind as well as your body. Certainly you're strengthening your cardiovascular system, which in itself will help prevent Alzheimer's, but you're using your brain, too.

Brain Aerobics and Einstein's Brain

Thinking exercises, a form of brain aerobics, have been reported to reduce your chance of developing Alzheimer's disease by 70 percent.

In a fascinating report, it was disclosed that the great thinker Albert Einstein, perhaps the most brilliant man in history, had normal brain cells (neurons). After his death, a famous pathologist examined the professor's brain and noted that his brain cells were the same as yours and mine. What was different was the supporting structure around his neurons, which showed a much higher level of development than usual. This supporting structure, similar to your skeleton, is referred to as glial cells. They support the connections between brain cells and are critically important.

The take-home message is that by thinking, you can improve these connections and thus enhance your memory. Some researchers believe that brain aerobics, especially combined with physical exercise such as walking, may actually regenerate brain cells. An innovative way to take advantage of this phenomenon is to combine physical exercise with brain aerobics.

Here's a fun idea: Go for a nice walk and sing your favorite song, or sing the national anthem as you jog—both will stimulate your memory. Another way to regenerate your brain cells is to ride an exercise bike, for example, and read a book at the same time. Or better yet, read the book and discuss it with a friend while you're exercising.

Michael, a 74-year-old man with multiple medical problems including Alzheimer's, used flash cards with his caregiver to beef up his memory. The cards featured movie stars from his era. Michael's caregiver would first do the mind/body exercises that I'll discuss with you in the next section. Then he would show him a card, for instance Marilyn Monroe, and ask who it was, what films she starred in, and other simple questions. The patient's family is sure that doing these exercises helped keep their loved one's Alzheimer's disease in check. Although Michael eventually passed away, it was from a cause unrelated to Alzheimer's.

In this kit I've created a set of memory exercise cards, each containing a special brain aerobic suggestion. Try a different one each day while you're participating in the other aspects of the program and see how much your memory improves.

Some Brain Aerobics

- Headline discussion
- Crossword and jigsaw puzzles
- Reading and discussing what you read
- Music, art, or other hobbies
- Learning a new language
- Becoming computer literate
- Shopping by memory (without a list)
- Volunteering
- Memorizing lists
- Discussing current events

Healing Your Brain with Mind/Body Exercises

The innovative exercises that I'm about to present to you are a fascinating example of the best principles of Asian medicine meeting the best Western medical research. For the past two decades, I've studied more than 2,000 of these techniques, which were taught to me by one of the leading yoga masters of our generation, Yogi Bhajan. Of those, I selected about 40 that were specifically developed to enhance memory function. I then used them in my clinical practice for the next 12 years. From the 40, I've selected the two easiest—yet most effective—memory-improving exercises to present to you. The first increases the amount of blood flow going to your brain, the second sends direct healing energy there, while both work to improve your memory. These techniques have clinically proven very useful over the years. Beyond that, *Kirtan Kriya,* the second one, has been tested in a research study.

Increasing Blood Flow to Your Brain

Although your brain makes up only 3 percent of your body weight, it receives 25 percent of the blood pumped by your heart. Sometimes, with age, people develop high cholesterol and arteriosclerosis, or hardening of the arteries. These conditions decrease the blood flow to your brain, thus increasing your risk for memory loss. That is why this first exercise is so important: It increases the amount of blood flow to your brain. The beautiful thing is that it only takes a few minutes to make it happen.

FIGURE 5

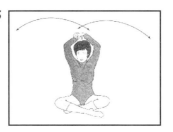

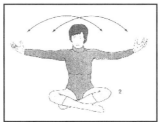

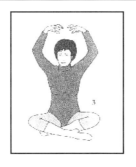

Instructions: Sit in a comfortable position on the floor or in a chair. Place your arms out to your sides, and make your hands into claws. Raise your arms up and cross them over your head (right over left and left over right). Repeat this motion breathing powerfully and rhythmically through the nose as demonstrated on the CD. Continue for three minutes, then inhale and thrust your tongue out as far as it will go and continue the movement for 15 more seconds. Exhale, and repeat. Then inhale and hold the position for 15 seconds. Exhale and relax by following the CD.

Next, follow the above exercise with Kirtan Kriya. This routine will supercharge your mind and memory.

Kirtan Kriya: Healing Your Brain and Improving Your Memory

Do you remember the four ingredients necessary to enter into the fourth state created by basic meditation? They are *comfort, quiet, a tool,* and *a special attitude,* which says to start all over again when other thoughts enter your mind and take the place of your tool. The mind/body exercise I'm about to share with you uses those same four steps. But it doesn't stop there—it also has five additional ingredients that give it immense power, precision, and practicality. The five new elements, in addition to the four original aspects of basic meditation, are as follows:

1. Breath
2. Posture
3. Healing sounds
4. Fingertip position
5. A unique focus of concentration

Kirtan Kriya, which means "a singing exercise complete in itself," is also popularly called "the five-primal-sounds meditation." The healing sounds in Kirtan Kriya are called the five primal sounds because they're the most healing tones in the universe, according to yogis. The sounds are: *Sa*, *Ta*, *Na*, and *Ma*. Sometimes people say, "But those are only four sounds." That is correct, but the *Ahh* at the end of each primal sound is common to all the sounds and thus is the fifth sound. In essence, it looks more like this: *Saa*, *Taa*, *Naa*, *Maa*.

In Kirtan Kriya, the breath comes naturally. You won't even have to think about it. All you have to do is inhale to begin and then follow the instructions on the CD.

The posture is simple. You can sit comfortably in a chair or cross-legged on the floor, in what we call *easy pose*. There's no difference in the result, as long as you sit up fairly straight.

Figure 6 on the next page shows how to do the meditation.

FIGURE 6

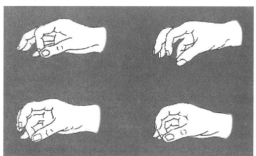
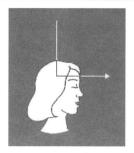
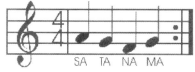

As you can see, when you chant the sound *Sa*, you touch your thumb to your index finger. When you say *Ta*, you touch your thumb to your middle finger. With *Na*, you touch your thumb to your ring finger. Finally, with *Ma*, your thumb and pinky touch.

You can see by the diagram that the L form of meditation is used as a focal point in Kirtan Kriya. As you chant each sound along with me on the CD, you imagine that it enters the top of your head and leaves through the middle of your forehead in a sweeping L motion. The movement is like a broom. From an energetic perspective, the sound is thus opening the channel between the top of your head, or seventh energy center of your body, which corresponds to your pineal gland, with the one corresponding with your pituitary gland, the sixth energy center.

The Science Behind Kirtan Kriya

When you touch your fingers to each other in succession as you chant the five primal sounds, a miraculous thing happens: Your brain becomes energized. This is because your fingers are highly represented in your brain. Since you pick up objects with your fingers, not your chest or stomach, the fingertips are very sensitive. In a map of the brain's touch receptors, called the homunculus, this is clear: Your fingers take up a large percentage of the map. So touching your fingers together not only serves to help induce a very relaxed state, it also activates your brain.

Singing or chanting the five primal sounds as directed has another incredible effect: Your brain chemistry is marvelously improved. Why is this so? Because, not unlike acupuncture points, which are located throughout your body, there are 54 points located on your upper palate or the roof of your mouth. Guess what's on the other side of your upper palate? If you said the master glands of your brain, the hypothalamus and pituitary glands, you go to the head of the class. Now, when you chant the sounds as directed on the CD, and your tongue touches the roof of your mouth, subtle energy in the form of sound vibrations is transmitted through your palate straight to your pituitary gland. The pituitary then orchestrates the release of healing chemicals that improve your memory. Not only that, but these chemicals are carried in your bloodstream to bring their many other health-giving effects to your whole being.

The following two pictures from the research project that I mentioned previously demonstrate the healing effects of Kirtan Kriya. Especially notice how chanting the primal sounds balances the brain.

FIGURE 7

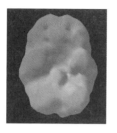 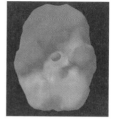

Before the meditation, notice the holes in the front part of the brain and the unevenness in the back part. Also, look at the flatness in the middle of the picture: This isn't a healthy brain. After the meditation, you can see that the holes are filled in signifying improved blood flow and energy. The back part of the brain is even, which brings the activities of the brain into balance. Finally, perhaps you can see the prominent 3-D dot rising up from the middle of the brain. This symbolizes a reduction in stress and tension, which improves memory.

When you complete the activities of the daily living chart in a later chapter, you'll decide when you want to practice the mind/body exercises. At that time, 8:00 A.M. for instance, simply use the CD and follow my lead. I know you're going to love it.

● ● ● ● ●

CHAPTER 12

The Power of Pharmaceutical Therapy

Delaying Alzheimer's

Early detection and prompt treatment of memory problems utilizing an integrative program, including drugs at the proper dose, may delay the development of Alzheimer's by many years. For that reason, I believe that there's a place for the use of pharmaceutical medications as part of an *integrative medical program* to prevent and treat Alzheimer's disease. Drugs are very useful, but they don't stand alone. To achieve the most favorable outcome, drugs used to prevent or treat Alzheimer's, and other forms of memory loss, must be combined with the other three pillars of *The Better Memory Kit*.

These medications should only be taken under the care of a physician who's an expert in treating Alzheimer's disease because all of these medicines may have serious side effects such as dizziness, nausea, diarrhea, and other symptoms.

The drugs currently in use are presented in order of preference:

1. Exelon® (rivastigmine): Start with 1.5 mg twice per day, proceeding to 3–6 mg twice per day. Exelon is slightly more effective than Aricept at slowing the rate of decline in a patient with Alzheimer's. This is because it blocks two chemical pathways, not just one, thus increasing the amount of memory chemicals in your brain. Exelon is probably most useful in people who are in the earliest stages of memory loss.

2. Reminyl® (galantamine): The starting dose is 4 mg twice per day, and may be increased to 8–12 mg twice per day, which is the most effective dosage range. Reminyl is the drug I mentioned that is derived from the nutrient galantamine. It increases the level of many different chemicals in your brain to help improve memory. It's most useful in patients with mid-stage to moderate Alzheimer's.

3. Aricept® (donepezil): 5–10 mg daily. Aricept, like Exelon, is moderately effective in improving short-term memory in patients with early Alzheimer's. One benefit of Aricept is that it may be taken only once a day in the morning, making it easier to use.

4. Namenda® (memantine): Usually started with 5 mg in the morning for two weeks, it's then often increased to a maximum of 40 mg per day slowly over a two-week period. Memantine has been available in many parts of the world for some time, and has had a modest effect in alleviating some of the symptoms of advanced Alzheimer's disease. According to a recent study, it has no significant side effects and was recently approved for use in the United States. The drug blocks a brain chemical called glutamate, which has been implicated in brain-cell death.

A St. Louis woman whose husband has advanced Alzheimer's disease, tells of trying memantine and having her husband remove a piece of chocolate coating from an ice cream bar and put it aside for her, as he used to do before he became ill. "This is for you," he told his wife. They're looking forward to more hopeful moments like this one.

If you recall, previously I discussed the horrible effects chronic stress has on your memory. One reason that chronic unbalanced stress kills brain cells by the thousands is because the hormone cortisol also disrupts glutamate function inside the brain. This disruption causes many free radicals to form inside your brain cells. It's interesting to note that memantine reverses that disruption and helps the brain.

That's why I'm so passionate about having you reduce your stress-induced cortisol levels with meditation. You can meditate now to prevent memory loss instead of waiting to take a drug when it's almost too late. This is a clear-cut case of the urgency and effectiveness of the preventive program presented in *The Better Memory Kit*.

Other Drugs

— Anti-Inflammatory Medicines (NSAIDs): 200 mg per day of ibuprofen (Advil, Motrin), clinoril (Sulindac), or indomethacin (Indocin). After two years of regular use at the proper dosage, NSAIDs may decrease your risk of Alzheimer's disease by 50 percent. NSAIDs should be taken with meals to reduce stomach irritation. NSAIDs do not reverse memory loss.

— **Aspirin (ASA):** 81 mg per day (1 baby aspirin). Aspirin deserves special mention because it may reduce your risk of developing Alzheimer's by as much as 55 percent. It also has a unique blood-thinning ability, which helps to prevent stroke and heart attacks.

Note: If you decide to take both an NSAID and ASA, alternate the days. **Do not** take them both on the same day.

— **Deprenyl:** An excellent drug, deprenyl, also called selegiline, has excellent antioxidant effects. Deprenyl also increases important brain chemicals. Patients of mine interested in optimal memory function, and memory-loss prevention and reversal have benefited from the use of deprenyl.

The dose of deprenyl varies but may start with as little as 3 mg per day. A breakthrough research study in Alzheimer's patients showed that 10 mg per day, combined with 2,000 IU per day of vitamin E, slowed the progression of the disease, allowing loved ones to stay at home rather than being placed into a nursing home.

— **Statins:** The dose depends on the drug used. Statins are used when you have high cholesterol not helped by diet and exercise. Elevated cholesterol is a risk factor for memory loss, including Alzheimer's disease. Statins may decrease the risk of developing memory loss by 79 percent to as much as 400 percent.

These drugs carry significant risks including muscle pain, muscle degeneration, and kidney failure, which can be fatal. One of the reasons for this side effect is that they cause the depletion of Coenzyme Q10. If you take statins, therefore, make sure that you also take *The Longevity Energy Caps,* which contain Coenzyme Q10.

The Red Yeast Story

One statin, Mevacor, contains the compound lovastatin. Lovastatin comes from red yeast extract. It's possible, therefore, that red yeast extract may reduce your risk of developing Alzheimer's at a much lower price than statin drugs. Red yeast extract comes in 600 mg capsules, and the usual dose is 2,400 mg per day. Two caps may be taken at dinner and two at bedtime, or if preferred, all four can be taken before you go to sleep. Your cholesterol and other lipids or blood fats should be checked after one month and your dose adjusted. Red yeast extract can be found at your health-food store.

Hormone Replacement Therapy (HRT)

Henry, a 75-year-old retired minister, attended one of our Better Memory seminars in Tucson. He was very ill. He had no energy, his memory was gone, and his diabetes was out of control. He couldn't breathe because of weakness and underlying lung disease. I measured his hormones and found them to be incredibly low, almost incompatible with life. I replaced the near-nonexistent levels of testosterone and DHEA, and he improved so fast that in a few weeks he was able to travel around the country, visiting friends and family he thought he was never going to see again.

There is strong clinical support to allow for careful HRT in people concerned about their memory. There are important considerations, however:

1. Hormone levels must be measured in the blood. If they're low, it makes sense to replace them in an informed manner. If they're not low, it's not safe to boost them higher than normal.

2. The hormone levels should be restored to the naturally occurring levels of a 30- to 40-year-old, and never younger.

3. Blood tests must be repeated every three months at first and then every six months to monitor hormone levels.

The hormones I measure include: DHEA, estrogen, progesterone, testosterone, and thyroid. Although I don't measure melatonin and pregnenolone, I replace them when clinically indicated. I know of no patient who has ever had a severe, life-threatening, or uncontrollable side effect from HRT. Beyond that, as a doctor experienced in its use, I can tell you that I've seen many people improve their memory, vitality, and their quality of life by replacing hormones when they're low.

Here's a brief description of each important hormone. Please see the chart that follows for the correct dose. (**Note:** hormones are powerful and can have side effects, which are best discussed with your doctor before beginning their use.)

Pregnenolone

Pregnenolone functions as a memory hormone. The brain even has specific receptors for it. One of my most gratifying professional experiences concerns the use of pregnenolone. In 1995, I was asked to see a 91-year-old woman with a Ph.D. in psychology. As amazing as it sounds, she was still practicing until she started losing her memory. She was deteriorating rapidly, and her family feared that she might have to go into an institution.

Pregnenolone came to this woman's rescue. I started her on a dose of 100 mg per day in concert with other aspects of this program. Her recovery was so dramatic that a local television station did a feature on her. She returned to being a part-time practicing psychologist and an elder in her church.

DHEA

I can count the number of patients suffering from memory loss who had normal levels of DHEA on one hand. I prescribe it extensively and have never been disappointed by its results. DHEA brings back the "juice of life." As with any other hormone, you should take DHEA under the supervision of your physician.

Estrogen

Reduced levels of estrogen have been related to an increased incidence of Alzheimer's disease. Estrogen use after menopause appears to reduce Alzheimer's risk by 50 percent. Use of this hormone in estrogen-deficient women can also help improve word recall.

Premarin, the estrogen-replacement drug most often utilized by conventional doctors, and the subject of hormone research, is composed of the urine of pregnant horses. Is that what you want to put in your body? A better choice is one of two natural forms of estrogen, Bi-est, a mixture of 80 percent estriol and 20 percent estradiol; or Tri-est, a balanced combination of 10 to 20 percent estradiol, 10 to 20 percent estrone, and 60 to 80 percent estriol. In contrast to unnatural Premarin, there's no difference in the composition of the natural hormones Bi-est and Tri-est with those produced by a woman's ovaries.

Progesterone

Natural progesterone is the forgotten player in HRT because many doctors ignore this quality-of-life–enhancing hormone. Replacing low levels of progesterone can make a big difference in a woman's total health, well-being, and mental function.

Testosterone

Maintaining youthful levels of testosterone is very important for the long-term health and vitality of both men and women. As low levels of this hormone may lead to short-term memory loss, as well as possibly increase Alzheimer's risk, replacing testosterone levels when they're low improves working memory and helps prevent Alzheimer's. The exact percentage of risk reduction with testosterone is not yet certain.

Thyroid Hormone

Among its many functions, the thyroid hormone regulates brain function. I always measure thyroid hormone levels in patients with memory complaints. Low levels, when replaced, may improve memory.

Melatonin

The amount of melatonin released by your pineal gland decreases with age, which creates sleeping difficulties in many patients. In order to have a good memory, you must sleep well. My patients who have a sleep problem are quite often pleased when I prescribe melatonin, for they say that it helps them sleep like they're 16 years old again. I've found that the dose required can vary widely: Some people need only a small dose, say ½ mg at bedtime, to get a good night's sleep, while others may need 3 mg or more. The correct dose is the amount that induces sleep rapidly, allows you to sleep through the night (ideally not even getting up to go to the bathroom), and permits you to wake up refreshed in the morning without feeling groggy. The exact percentage of Alzheimer's risk reduction is not yet certain.

By following the Better Memory program, you'll need less supplemental melatonin as you restore the health of your brain.

Measuring Blood Levels of Hormones

Following is the list of blood tests I recommend to measure hormone levels, their normal values, and replacement dosages. The name of the hormone is listed in bold, followed by the lab values, then the treatment. *Please note:* Lab values may vary according to laboratory.

FIGURE 8

DHEA Men
Lab values: 146–850
Treatment: 25–100 mg per day

DHEA Women
Lab values: 112–722
Treatment: 25–100 mg per day

Free Testosterone Men
Lab values: 7.2–24
Treatment: 10–50 mg in a cream applied once or twice per day

Free Testosterone Women
Lab values: Premenopausal: 1.1–8.5
Treatment: 2–8 mg in a cream applied once or twice per day

Lab values: Postmenopausal: 0.6–6.7
Treatment: 2–8 mg in a cream applied once or twice per day

TSH (Marker of Thyroid)
Lab values: 0.35–500
Treatment: ½ grain–3 grains per day

Free T3 (Thyroid Hormone)
Lab values: 2.3–4.2
Treatment: See TSH

Free T4 (Thyroid Hormone)
Lab values: 0.70–1.53
Treatment: See TSH

Estradiol (Estrogen)
Lab values: 25–443
Treatment: Bi-Est 2.5–5 mg per day; Tri-Est 2.5–5 mg per day

(Cont'd. on next page)

FIGURE 8, cont'd.

Progesterone
Lab values: 150–300
Treatment: 100–300 mg twice per day

Melatonin
Lab values: Not usually measured
Treatment: 1 mg–3 mg for sleep

Pregnenolone
Lab values: Not usually measured
Treatment: 10–100 mg per day

CHAPTER 13

7 Days to a Better Memory

The famous Chinese philosopher Lao-tzu once wrote: "A journey of a thousand miles begins with a single step." I predict that you'll come to consider this moment a turning point in your life, because now you'll take your first step toward building a better memory. Many of my patients feel this way because this is the time when you begin actively designing your own personalized better memory program.

You'll notice a difference in how your memory works almost immediately. For example, Bob, a 55-year-old pastor and psychotherapist from New Mexico, was suffering greatly from low mental energy, inability to remember the names of members of his congregation, and difficulty recalling phone numbers. His mother had died from Alzheimer's, and he was afraid he was in the early stages of the disease. I was worried, too, because all his tests were pointing in that direction.

I designed a full-spectrum Better Memory program for Bob, and after the first day he noticed a remarkable improvement. How could that be? For one thing, I felt that Bob was deficient in B vitamins and therefore supplementing his diet with my high-potency *Longevity Gold Caps,* which are rich in B's, gave him an immediate boost of energy. Furthermore, I thought he had poor circulation to his brain. Taking Ginkgo Biloba and doing the mind/body exercises brought new life to him, as it drove blood to places deep in his brain where it hadn't been in years. I remember him saying, "Dr. Dharma, it feels like I haven't had this much oxygen to my brain in 20 years."

Within seven days, Bob was functioning

at a whole new level and was very happy with his progress. He continued on the program and enjoyed further improvement in his energy, concentration, and learning abilities.

Many other patients of mine are also seeing rapid improvement. One thing that I've noticed is that the more a person needs the program, the faster the response. Of course, I recommend that you continue with the program even if your improvement isn't as fast or as dramatic as Bob's. Virtually everyone does respond; some simply take a little longer. But in the first week of participating in the program, you'll begin replenishing your brain with nutrients it lacks, increasing the oxygen to your memory center, and enhancing your mental energy. You'll begin to build a habit pattern that will serve you well for the rest of your life.

The charts that I provide in this chapter will give you everything you need to design your own program, which is divided into five sections:

1. Optimizing Memory and Preventing Alzheimer's
2. Mild Cognitive Impairment (MCI)
3. Early-Stage Alzheimer's
4. Mid- to Late-Stage Alzheimer's
5. Special Circumstances: Adult ADD, chronic fatigue, chemo-brain

Class 1: Optimizing Memory and Preventing Alzheimer's

1. Diet: Follow a 15 to 20 percent right-fat diet as described previously. Consider consulting a nutritionist. Eat free-range beef, chicken, and nonfarmed fish. Have at least seven servings of organic fruit and vegetables daily. Make your shopping cart (and plate) a beautiful rainbow of nutrition. Use alcohol sparingly.

2. Stress Management: Pay attention to your stressors. See how you can simplify your life. Follow the CD for meditation. Stop and take a few deep breaths throughout the day. Take a yoga or Pilates class.

3. Physical Exercise: You should exercise four times a week, working at up to 80 percent of your aerobic capacity, if possible. You can determine your aerobic capacity with the following formula: 220-age x .80 = heartbeats per minute. For example, if you're 60 years old: 220-60 = 160 x .80 = 128 beats per minute. Strength training is also excellent.

4. Mind/Body Exercise: Start each day in a positive way. Set yourself right each morning with the mind/body exercises on the CD. Use the *Sleepy-Time Nice* (Track 3) at night if needed.

5. Brain Aerobics: Please begin to take cognitive exercise seriously. Discover new ways to exercise your mind. Follow the instructions for using the memory exercise cards, and create your own type of mental exercises or stories. Use the cards three times a week. Engage a friend or significant other to do them with you. You'll both benefit.

6. Vitamins and Memory-Specific Nutrients: Optimizing/Preventing

FIGURE 9

Longevity Gold Caps
Dosage: 3 with breakfast & 3 with lunch

Longevity Brain Tabs
Dosage: 2 with breakfast
Comment: May add 2 with lunch if needed

Longevity Memory Caps
Dosage: None

Longevity Energy Caps
Dosage: 1 with breakfast

Longevity Green Drink
Dosage: ½ scoop in a morning drink or smoothie
Comment: If you need extra energy

> **Longevity Prostate Caps**
> *Dosage:* 1 with breakfast, 1 with lunch, & 1 with dinner
> *Comment:* For males over 45, especially if taking DHEA or Testosterone

7. Hormones: Optimizing /Preventing

> **FIGURE 10**
>
> **DHEA**
> *Dosage:* 25–100 mg /day with breakfast
> Dose depends on sex, age, and blood level
> *Comment:* I use compounded DHEA. It should be monitored by a physician
>
> **Pregnenolone**
> *Dosage:* 10–100 mg per day with breakfast, or according to your physician
> *Comment:* I use compounded Pregnenolone; I rarely use it in prevention and hardly ever in combination with DHEA
>
> (Cont'd. on next page)

FIGURE 10, cont'd.

Melatonin
Dosage: ⅓–3 mg at bed time, or as prescribed by your physician
Comment: I usually use a compounding pharmacy

Estrogen
Dosage: As per chart in Chapter 9
Comment: Bi-est or tri-est (natural estrogen) and as prescribed by your doctor

Progesterone
Dosage: As per chart in Chapter 9
Comment: As prescribed by your doctor

Testosterone
Dosage: As per chart in Chapter 9
Comment: As prescribed by your doctor

8. Pharmaceuticals: Optimizing/Preventing

— **Deprenyl:** 1–3 mg per day from a compounding pharmacy. Should be used under a physician's care. May not be needed at this point, especially if you follow the other aspects of the program. No negative interaction with drugs described below but should **NEVER** be used with the **MAO-I** class of antidepressants. Reaction could be fatal.

— **Aricept, Exelon, Reminyl, Memantine:** Not indicated at this level.

— **Anti-inflammatories:** See Chapter 8.

Comments: The best time to institute a Better Memory program is before you begin noticing that your memory isn't working as well as it used to.

Class 2: Mild Cognitive Impairment (MCI)

1. Diet: Eat very little saturated fat. This means effectively eliminating red meat. I suggest that you get your protein exclusively from seafood such as fresh-frozen Alaskan salmon or tuna-fish steak (as opposed to canned tuna). Make a rainbow plate of fresh, lightly steamed organic vegetables the mainstay of your diet. Try the Tucson Power Plate recipe (see page 84). No alcohol should be taken.

2. Stress Management: Make meditation the key ingredient of your reduced-stress lifestyle. It's the most crucial element and the one quite often overlooked. Do it every afternoon. Think about how to reduce the demands placed on you.

3. Physical Exercise: Working out will help keep you from progressing to Alzheimer's. Join a gym and hire a trainer. Walk, walk, and walk some more.

4. Mind/Body: Don't miss a day of the morning mind/body exercises on the CD for one month.

5. Brain Aerobics: A good time for mental exercise is after physical or mind/body exercise. Use the cards at least four times a week.

6. Vitamins and Memory-Specific Nutrients: MCI

FIGURE 11

Longevity Gold Caps
Dosage: 3 with breakfast & 3 with lunch

Longevity Brain Tabs
Dosage: 2 with breakfast & 2 with lunch

Longevity Memory Caps
Dosage: 1 with breakfast
Comment: May add 1 cap with lunch, depending on symptoms

(Cont d. on next page)

FIGURE 11, cont'd.

Longevity Energy Caps
Dosage: 1 with breakfast

Longevity Green Drink
Dosage: ½ scoop with morning juice,
water, or smoothie

Longevity Prostate Caps
Dosage: 1 with breakfast,
1 with lunch & 1 with dinner
Comment: For males over 45, especially if
taking DHEA or testosterone

Galantamine
Comment: Nutrient may be
preferred over drugs in MCI

Note: Make sure your total dose of vitamin E is at least 1,000 IU and preferably 2,000 IU.

7. Hormones: MCI

FIGURE 12

DHEA

Dosage: 25–100 mg /day with breakfast. Dose depends on sex, age, and blood level

Comments: I use compounded DHEA. Should be monitored by a physician

Pregnenolone

Dosage: 10–100 mg per day at breakfast or according to your physician

Comments: I use compounded Pregnenolone. May be very useful in MCI, especially in women

Melatonin

Dosage: 1/3–3 mg at bedtime as prescribed by your physician

Comments: I usually use a compounding pharmacy

(Cont'd. on next page)

FIGURE 12, cont'd.

Estrogen
Dosage: As per chart in Chapter 9
Comments: Bi-est or tri-est (natural estrogen) and as prescribed by your doctor

Progesterone
Dosage: As per chart in Chapter 9
Comments: As prescribed by your doctor

Testosterone
Dosage: As per chart in Chapter 9
Comments: As prescribed by your doctor

8. Pharmaceuticals: MCI. Remember, no drug stands alone. When implementing drug therapy in MCI, you'll achieve the best results using a combined integrative medical approach.

— **Deprenyl:** 5–10 mg per day as prescribed by your doctor. I use a compounding pharmacy. No negative interaction with drugs described below but should **NEVER** be used with the **MAO-I** class of antidepressants drugs. The reaction could be fatal.

— **Exelon:** First choice in treating MCI if a drug is used. See the chart in Chapter 9 and follow your doctor's instructions as you increase the dose.

— **Aricept:** Not a first choice.

— **Reminyl:** Nutrient Galantamine is probably a better choice than Reminyl for MCI.

— **Memantine:** Not used for MCI.

— **Anti-inflammatories:** See Chapter 8.

Comments: With early diagnosis and treatment using an integrative medical approach, we can prevent MCI from progressing to Alzheimer's.

Class 3: Early-Stage Alzheimer's Disease

1. Diet: Eat very little saturated fat. This means effectively eliminating red meat. I suggest that you get your protein exclusively from fish such as fresh-frozen Alaskan salmon or tuna-fish steak (as opposed to canned tuna). Make a rainbow plate of fresh lightly steamed organic vegetables the mainstay of your diet. No alcohol should be taken.

2. Stress Management: The CD must be used to practice meditation every day without fail. The best time will be determined in the next chapter. Because of memory loss, stress is increased and cortisol is high. Therefore, meditation is critical. If concentration proves too difficult for meditation, play relaxing music or sing familiar songs. Watching home videos is also comforting.

3. Physical Exercise: People with early Alzheimer's are able to exercise, especially with a personal trainer or assistant. It's important to keep moving and walking.

4. Mind/Body: With assistance, the mind/body exercise part of the CD can still be accomplished. It helps increase brain energy and organizational skills.

5. Brain Aerobics: While some functional loss may inhibit the ability to practice meditation or various exercises, brain aerobics are imperative. Set a daily time according to the chart in the next chapter for the patient and caregiver or loved one to use the flash cards.

6. Vitamins and Memory-Specific Nutrients: Early Alzheimer's

FIGURE 13

Longevity Gold Caps
Dosage: 3 with breakfast & 3 with lunch

Longevity Brain Tabs
Dosage: 2 with breakfast, 2 with lunch & 2 with dinner

Longevity Memory Caps
Dosage: 1 with breakfast & 1 with lunch

Longevity Energy Caps
Dosage: 1 with breakfast

Longevity Green Drink
Dosage: ½ scoop with morning juice, water, or smoothie for energy
Comments: Optional

Longevity Prostate Caps
Dosage: 1 cap with breakfast, 1 with lunch & 1 with dinner
Comments: For males over 45, especially if taking DHEA or Testosterone

> **Galantamine**
> *Comments:* Drug Reminyl preferred at this stage

Note: Make sure your total dose of vitamin E is 2,000 IU.

7. Hormones: Early Alzheimer's

> **FIGURE 14**
>
> **DHEA**
> *Dosage:* 25–100 mg /day with breakfast. Dose depends on sex, age, and blood level
> *Comments:* I use compounded DHEA. It should be monitored by a physician
>
> **Pregnenolone**
> *Dosage:* 10–100 mg per day at breakfast according to your physician
> *Comments:* I use compounded Pregnenolone
>
> (Cont'd. on next page)

FIGURE 14, cont'd.

Melatonin
Dosage: ⅓–3 mg at bedtime as prescribed by your physician
Comments: I usually use a compounding pharmacy

Estrogen
Dosage: As per chart in Chapter 9
Comments: Bi-est or tri-est (natural estrogen) and as prescribed by your doctor

Progesterone
Dosage: As per chart in Chapter 9
Comments: As prescribed by your doctor

Testosterone
Dosage: As per chart in Chapter 9
Comments: As prescribed by your doctor

8. Pharmaceuticals: Early Alzheimer's. Remember, no drug stands alone. You'll achieve the best results using a combined integrative medical approach.

— **Deprenyl:** 5–10 mg per day as prescribed by your doctor. I use a compounding pharmacy. No negative interaction with drugs described below but should **NEVER** be used with the **MAO-I** class of antidepressants. Reaction could be fatal.

— **Exelon:** First choice in early Alzheimer's. See the chart in Chapter 9 and follow your doctor's instructions as you increase the dose.

— **Aricept:** Not a first choice, but may improve function for a period of time.

— **Reminyl:** May be useful in conjunction with Exelon. See the chart in Chapter 9 for dose. Follow your doctor's instructions.

— **Memantine:** Not used in early Alzheimer's.

— **Anti-inflammatories:** Won't slow progression but will prevent stroke and heart attack.

Comments: It's realistic to expect to improve function and delay progression in early Alzheimer's disease.

Class 4: Mid- to Late-Stage Alzheimer's

1. Diet: Eat very little saturated fat. This means effectively eliminating red meat. I suggest you get your protein exclusively from fish such as fresh-frozen Alaskan salmon or tuna-fish steak (as opposed to canned tuna). Make a rainbow plate of fresh lightly steamed organic vegetables the mainstay of your diet. No alcohol should be taken.

2. Stress Management: At this stage, meditation is difficult. Listening to one's favorite music, singing familiar songs, and watching home videos reduces stress.

3. Physical Exercise: People with Alzheimer's may not be able to exercise because of memory loss and balance difficulty. Physical therapy and therapeutic massage serve a useful purpose at this stage.

4. Mind/Body: It's difficult to do mind/body exercises at this stage but worth the effort with assistance. Will help with orientation.

5. Brain Aerobics: Brain aerobics are imperative to maintain as much function as possible and delay further progression. Set a daily time according to the chart in the next chapter for the patient and caregiver or loved one to use the cards or make up brain games.

6. Vitamins and Memory-Specific Nutrients: Mid- to Late-Stage Alzheimer's

FIGURE 15

Longevity Gold Caps
Dosage: 3 with breakfast & 3 with lunch

Longevity Brain Tabs
Dosage: 2 with breakfast, 2 with lunch & 2 with dinner

Longevity Memory Caps
Dosage: 1 with breakfast & 1 with lunch

Longevity Energy Caps
Dosage: 1 with breakfast

Longevity Green Drink
Dosage: ½ scoop with morning juice, water, or smoothie for energy
Comments: Optional

Longevity Prostate Caps
Dosage: 1 with breakfast, 1 with lunch & 1 with dinner
Comments: For males over 45, especially if taking DHEA or Testosterone

Galantamine
Comments: Drug Reminyl preferred at this stage

Note: Make sure your total dose of Vitamin E is 2,000 IU.

7. Hormones: Mid- to Late-Stage Alzheimer's

FIGURE 16

DHEA
Dosage: 25–100 mg /day with breakfast. Dose depends on sex, age, and blood level
Comments: I use compounded DHEA. It should be monitored by a physician

Pregnenolone
Dosage: 10–100 mg per day at breakfast according to your physician
Comments: I use compounded Pregnenolone

(Cont'd. on next page)

FIGURE 16, cont'd.

Melatonin
Dosage: ⅓–3 mg at bedtime as prescribed by your physician
Comments: I usually use a compounding pharmacy

Estrogen
Dosage: As per chart in Chapter 9
Comments: Bi-est or tri-est (natural estrogen) and as prescribed by your doctor

Progesterone
Dosage: As per chart in Chapter 9
Comments: As prescribed by your doctor

Testosterone
Dosage: As per chart in Chapter 9
Comments: As prescribed by your doctor

8. Pharmaceuticals: Mid- to Late-Stage Alzheimer's.

It's still possible to maintain a certain level of function and slow progression of the disease. You'll achieve the best results using a combined integrative medical approach.

— **Deprenyl:** 5–10 mg per day as prescribed by your doctor. I use a compounding pharmacy. No negative interaction with drugs described below but should **NEVER** be used with the **MAO-I** class of antidepressants. Reaction could be fatal.

— **Exelon:** First choice for this stage. See chart in Chapter 9 and follow your doctor's instructions as you increase the dose.

— **Aricept:** Not a first choice, but may improve function for a period of time.

— **Reminyl:** Probably not indicated at this stage.

— **Memantine:** This drug *is* useful at this stage. It may improve balance, speech, and fine motor skills. See Chapter 9 and work with your doctor.

— **Anti-inflammatories:** Won't affect progression of disease but may prevent heart attack or stroke.

Comments: By following an integrative program, it's possible to have the patient with mid- to late-stage disease maintain dignity. We can improve many symptoms and slow the progression.

Special Circumstances: Adult ADD, Chronic Fatigue, Chemo-Brain

1. Diet: Follow a 15 to 20 percent good-fat diet as described in Chapter 8. Consider consulting a nutritionist. Eat free-range beef, chicken, and nonfarmed fish. Have at least seven servings of organic fruit and vegetables daily. Make your shopping cart (and plate) a beautiful rainbow of nutrition. Use alcohol sparingly.

2. Stress Management: Meditation is your magic bullet.

3. Physical Exercise: Graded exercise has been proven to increase energy and mental function in these situations. Experiment and discover where you develop fatigue and exercise up to right before that point. You'll find that it will change as you increase your endurance.

4. Mind/Body Exercise: Start each day in a positive way. The mind/body exercises on the CD will provide great energy, attention, and focus.

5. Brain Aerobics: Discover new ways to exercise your mind. Follow the instructions for using the memory exercise cards, and create your own type of mental exercises or stories.

6. Vitamins and Memory-Specific Nutrients: Special Circumstances

FIGURE 17

Longevity Gold Caps
Dosage: 3 with breakfast & 3 with lunch

Longevity Brain Tabs
Dosage: 2 with breakfast & 2 with lunch, & 2 with dinner

Longevity Memory Caps
Dosage: 1 with breakfast & 1 with lunch
Comments: Optional. Needs to be individualized. Work with your doctor.

Longevity Energy Caps
Dosage: 1 with breakfast

Longevity Green Drink
Dosage: ½ scoop with morning juice, water, or smoothie for energy
Comments: Excellent for energy in these circumstances

Longevity Prostate Caps
Dosage: 1 with breakfast, 1 with lunch, & 1 with dinner
Comment: For males over 45, especially if taking DHEA or testosterone

7. Hormones: Special Circumstances

FIGURE 18

DHEA
Dosage: 25–100 mg /day with breakfast
Dose depends on sex, age, and blood level
Comments: I use compounded DHEA. It should be monitored by a physician. Research shows benefit in chronic fatigue.

Pregnenolone
Dosage: 10–100 mg per day at breakfast according to your physician
Comments: I use compounded Pregnenolone. May be useful in these cases.

(Cont'd. on next page)

FIGURE 18, cont'd.

Melatonin
Dosage: ⅓–3 mg at bedtime as prescribed by your physician
Comments: I usually use a compounding pharmacy

Estrogen
Dosage: As per chart in Chapter 9
Comments: Bi-est or tri-est (natural estrogen) and as prescribed by your doctor

Progesterone
Dosage: As per chart in Chapter 9
Comments: As prescribed by your doctor

Testosterone
Dosage: As per chart in Chapter 9
Comments: As prescribed by your doctor

8. Pharmaceuticals: Special Circumstances

— **Deprenyl:** 1–3 mg per day from a compounding pharmacy. Should be taken under a physician's care. May be helpful depending on age and function. No negative interaction with drugs described below but should **NEVER** be used with the **MAO-I** class of antidepressants. Reaction could be fatal.

— **Aricept, Exelon, Reminyl, Memantine:** Not indicated.

— **Anti-inflammatories:** Not indicated for memory. May prevent heart attack and stroke at lower doses and decrease pain in higher doses.

Comments: This program will increase your energy and improve your memory function.

CHAPTER 14

Creating Your Own Personal Better Memory Program

Congratulations! You've worked very hard to get to this point in the kit, and now comes the payoff. In this chapter, you'll plug your Better Memory program actions into your daily activities. Below is a sample schedule. Study it and then complete your own schedule.

I've also included a very special visualization on the CD to help you clarify how you'll incorporate the program into your lifestyle. Please do that exercise before continuing in this booklet. As you prepare to do the visualization, which you may repeat

often, please consider the following.
In your mind's eye:

1. Think back to a time when you completed a goal successfully.

2. Think of what you've learned so far, and what you need to do now to meet your goal of developing a better memory.

3. Finally, see what the successful completion of your goal looks like in the future. How does it feel to successfully complete the program found in *The Better Memory Kit?*

After completing this visualization on the CD, please return to this spot in your booklet. Here's a synopsis of the general aspects of the program:

— **Diet:** Eat well. Smaller portion sizes, lower fat (but right fats), rich in omega-3 oils. Good carbohydrates and solid protein.

Limit saturated fat from animal products. Take vitamins and memory supplements as prescribed.

— **Stress Management:** Daily afternoon meditation.

— **Exercise:** *Physical:* Three to four times a week. *Mental:* Three evenings a week. *Mind/Body:* A great way to start every day.

— **Pharmaceuticals:** Drugs and hormones as needed.

Sample Daily Schedule

6:00 A.M.	Wake up, shower, etc.
6:30 A.M.	Mind/body exercises on CD
7:00 A.M.	Breakfast, take vitamins, nutrients, and/or drugs
8:00 A.M.	Leave for work

9:00 A.M.	Arrive at work
10:00 A.M.	Take Deprenyl; work until lunch
12:00 (Noon)	Lunch/vitamins, nutrients, etc.
1:00–5:00 P.M.	Working (take a relaxation, stretch, or walking break if possible)
5:00 P.M.	Go to gym for exercise three days a week
6:45 P.M.	Arrive home
7:00 P.M.	Short meditation
7:30 P.M.	Dinner

After dinner three evenings a week, engage in brain aerobics using memory exercise cards. This is an excellent opportunity for quality family time. You can watch television on other days.

10:00 P.M. Time for sleep. May use *Sleepy-Time Nice* meditation (Track 3) to help you ease into a peaceful night's sleep.

Better Memory Reminder

- Can you find the time to do your morning mind/body exercises?
- Can you modify your diet?
- Will you make sure you take the vitamins, nutrients, and drugs/hormones?
- When can you do physical exercises?
- Will you fit in an afternoon meditation?
- Can you do brain aerobics at regular times?

My Daily Activity Schedule

6:00 A.M.

7:00 A.M.

8:00 A.M.

9:00 A.M.

10:00 A.M.

11:00 A.M.

12:00 (Noon)

1:00 P.M.

2:00 P.M.

3:00 P.M.

4:00 P.M.

5:00 P.M.

6:00 P.M.

7:00 P.M.

8:00 P.M.

9:00 P.M.

10:00 P.M.

CHAPTER 15

The Final Frontier

Wisdom, Beauty, and Life Satisfaction

Sociological research tells us that life satisfaction does not depend on financial assets, social status, or physical environment. Rather, it's conditional on what I call *applied intelligence,* which is the useful combination of knowledge, experience, and reflection. Applied intelligence gives you the capacity to make choices based on your higher or spiritual values rather than choosing to follow your emotions, addictions, or insecurities. Satisfaction with life, it seems, is as much about how well you know yourself and how much you give to others as it is about what you have.

One of my favorite sayings is by the

beloved writer Ralph Waldo Emerson, who wrote: "What lies behind us and what lies before us are tiny matters compared to what lies within us." It is my deepest hope and prayer that by using this kit you'll enjoy many years of great memory. But equally important is my hope that you use this time of heightened cognition to look within and discover your own true identity. My experience is that when you do so, you'll realize your own divine essence, and that will bring you the greatest happiness you could ever have.

Remember, you're not a human being searching for spirit. You are, instead, a spiritual being having a human experience.

My ultimate purpose in doing this work is to help you keep your mind alive forever. My prayer is that you develop applied intelligence so that you can share your great wisdom with your family, your friends, and your community to benefit the greater good. In this way, perhaps we can help make this world a better place for those who come after us.

This kit is only the beginning. As the saying goes: "Today is the first day of the rest of your life."

● ● ● ● ●

ACKNOWLEDGMENTS

Thanks to my agent, Mr. Richard Pine, of Arthur Pine and Associates, for working with me to find the absolute right home for this project. Also thanks to Reid Tracy, president/CEO of Hay House, for his creative vision. Jill, my editor; and Christy, my art director, did a fantastic job from day one. Stacey Smith, Reid's assistant, was always there and very helpful.

A special acknowledgment to my lovely wife, Kirti Khalsa, COO and cofounder and secretary of the Board of Directors of the Alzheimer's Prevention Foundation International (APFI); Randal Brooks, vice president; Carolyn Sechler, CPA, treasurer; and Carolyn Lucz, member of the APFI Board of Directors. I'd like to offer my appreciation to Nisha Money, M.D., chair of the APFI's research committee, as well as to Daniel Amen, M.D.; Chris Hanks, Ph.D.; Rod Shankel, M.D.; and Yogesh Shah, M.D., for their help with our research projects.

Also my appreciation goes to Martin Zamora, my right-hand man, as well as Alison Miller, Terry Gossell, and Peggy Smith of the APFI.

I'm grateful for the support, friendship, and partnership of Leeza Gibbons, founder, and Jamie Huysman, LCSW, executive director, of the Leeza Gibbons Memory Foundation. I'd also like to express my appreciation to Eric Hall, CEO, and Carol Steinberg, vice president of The Alzheimer's Foundation of America, for our friendship, affiliation, and work together to help end Alzheimer's disease.

Special mention goes to Somers White, C.P.A.E., my business mentor for close to two decades. Somers has handled more than 30 assignments for me, all with superb results.

I'm grateful to have Jo Cavender of Speakers Connection as my speaking agent.

I'd like to offer a special thanks to M.S.S. Livtar Singh Khalsa, affectionately known as Master L, for helping in the creation and production of the CD.

Finally, I send my appreciation to Louise Hay for creating Hay House. You do a great service for humanity.

— **Dharma Singh Khalsa, M.D.**
Tucson, Arizona

RESOURCES

To learn more about the work of Dharma Singh Khalsa, M.D., purchase the products recommended in *The Better Memory Kit,* view Dr. Dharma's speaking schedule, book a consultation, or attend a Better Memory seminar or workshop, please visit this Website: **www.drdharma.com**. And you may also purchase the products by calling (888) 234-0459.

We will also be able to serve you online by offering:

- Recipes
- Weekly online meetings with Q&A's
- Live-chat auditoriums with Dr. Dharma and other experts
- Chat rooms for sharing ideas and experiences

- Expert advice
- Seminars
- Consultations
- A newsletter

To explore having Dharma Singh Khalsa, M.D., speak for your group, please visit: **www.speakersconnection.com**.

You may also contact him through:

Jo Cavender
Speakers Connection
514 N.W. 11th Ave., Ste. 209
Portland, OR 97209
(800) 697-7325

Alzheimer's Foundation of America (AFA)
Eric Hall, CEO
322 8th Ave., 6th Floor
New York, NY 10001
(866) AFA-8484
e-mail: info@alzfdn.org
www.alzfdn.org

The AFA is a nonprofit foundation comprised of member and associate member organizations across the United States dedicated to meeting the educational, social, and emotional needs of individuals with Alzheimer's disease, their families, and caregivers. The AFA also strives to raise public awareness about the disease and lends expertise to health-care professionals. The AFA is the home of the first Leeza's Place in the U.S.

Alzheimer's Prevention Foundation International (APFI)
Dharma Singh Khalsa, M.D.
President/Medical Director
2420 N. Pantano Road
Tucson, AZ 85715
(520) 749-8374
Fax: (520) 296-6640
e-mail: info@AlzheimersPrevention.org
www.AlzheimersPrevention.org

APFI is a 501(c)(3) charitable organization working to reduce the incidence of Alzheimer's disease through clinical research, advocacy, and educational outreach. It's dedicated to the prevention of early memory loss and Alzheimer's disease.

The foundation's mission is to make available research results and the latest information, from both conventional and alternative or complementary medicine, to empower individuals and their families to nurture the health of their brains . . . and to give them hope. APFI is the original voice of Alzheimer's prevention.

Leeza Gibbons Memory Foundation and Leeza's Place

James Huysman, LCSW
Executive Director
3050 Biscayne Boulevard, Suite 908
Miami, Florida 33137
(888) OK-Leeza
www.leezasplace.org

The Leeza Gibbons Memory Foundation was created to fulfill Leeza's promise to her mother when her mom was diagnosed with Alzheimer's. The foundation's mission includes helping caregivers take better care of their patients and loved ones who suffer from Alzheimer's disease and other forms of memory loss.

Leeza's Place is an intimate and safe setting where caregivers and those recently diagnosed with any neurological disorder can gather to prepare themselves for the challenging journey ahead. There they will find the three cornerstones of Leeza's Place: empowerment, education, and energy.

● ● ● ● ●

If you'd like to see the medical references for this program, please visit: **www.drdharma.com**.

● ● ● ● ●

ABOUT THE AUTHOR

Born in Ohio and raised in Florida, **Dharma Singh Khalsa, M.D.,** is the world's leading expert on the integrative medical approach to the prevention of Alzheimer's disease, and he's the first doctor to testify before Congress on this topic. After his testimony, Dr. Khalsa received the support of the U.S. Surgeon General.

Dr. Khalsa is the president/medical director of the Alzheimer's Prevention Foundation International (APFI) in Tucson, Arizona. The APFI is the original voice of Alzheimer's prevention in the medical community.

Dharma has written four best-selling books, authored numerous articles in the lay press, and several chapters on Alzheimer's disease in medical textbooks. He has also created ten CDs and an audiotape (*Meditations for Healing*) with Deepak Chopra, M.D. He lectures and consults worldwide.

To learn more about the work of Dr. Dharma Singh Khalsa, M.D., visit: **www.drdharma.com**.

MORE KITS AVAILABLE FROM HAY HOUSE

The Best Year of Your Life Kit,
by Debbie Ford (available January 2005)

Connecting with Your Angels Kit,
by Doreen Virtue, Ph.D.

The Detox Kit, by Jane Alexander

8 Minutes in the Morning Kit,
by Jorge Cruise

The Good Night Sleep Kit, by Deepak Chopra, M.D. (available April 2005)

You Can Heal Your Life Affirmation Kit,
by Louise L. Hay

All of the above are available at your local bookstore, or may be ordered by contacting Hay House.

We hope you enjoyed this Hay House Lifestyles guidebook. If you would like to receive a free catalog featuring additional Hay House books and products, or if you would like information about the Hay Foundation, please contact:

Hay House, Inc.
P.O. Box 5100
Carlsbad, CA 92018-5100
(760) 431-7695 or **(800) 654-5126**
(760) 431-6948 (fax) or **(800) 650-5115 (fax)**
www.hayhouse.com

• • • • •

Published and distributed in Australia by: Hay House Australia Pty. Ltd. • 18/36 Ralph St. • Alexandria NSW 2015 • *Phone:* 612-9669-4299 • *Fax:* 612-9669-4144 • www.hayhouse.com.au

Published and distributed in the United Kingdom by: Hay House UK, Ltd. • Unit 62, Canalot Studios 222 Kensal Rd., London W10 5BN • *Phone:* 44-20-8962-1230 • *Fax:* 44-20-8962-1239 • www.hayhouse.co.uk

Published and distributed in the Republic of South Africa by: Hay House SA (Pty), Ltd., P.O. Box 990, Witkoppen 2068 • *Phone/Fax:* 2711-7012233
orders@psdprom.co.za

Distributed in Canada by: Raincoast • 9050 Shaughnessy St., Vancouver, B.C. V6P 6E5 • *Phone:* (604) 323-7100 • *Fax:* (604) 323-2600

⁕ ⁕ ⁕ ⁕ ⁕

Sign up via the Hay House USA Website to receive the Hay House online newsletter and stay informed about what's going on with your favorite authors. You'll receive bimonthly announcements about: Discounts and Offers, Special Events, Product Highlights, Free Excerpts, Giveaways, and more!
www.hayhouse.com

⁕ ⁕ ⁕ ⁕ ⁕